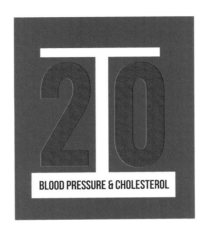

BLOOD PRESSURE & CHOLESTEROL

DR. FUHRMAN'S TRANSFORMATION 20 BLOOD PRESSURE & CHOLESTEROL
SIGNIFICANTLY LOWER YOUR BLOOD PRESSURE AND CHOLESTEROL IN 20 DAYS WITHOUT DRUGS

Joel Fuhrman, M.D.

Published by:
Gift of Health Press

FOREWORD

I am pleased to offer you the opportunity to transform your health and significantly lower your blood pressure and cholesterol. A diagnosis of high blood pressure or high cholesterol is a serious issue that should not be ignored, as it reflects a heightened risk of heart attack and stroke. Superior nutrition is the most effective remedy, but it is often disregarded because it isn't as easy as taking a pill. Evidence and clinical experience suggest that nutritional excellence is a hundred times more effective at preventing future heart attacks and strokes compared to drugs. In this booklet, I give you the most effective prescription for obtaining optimal health.

By eating a Nutritarian (nutrient-dense, plant-rich) diet, you can achieve better blood pressure readings and cholesterol levels than you have had in years. It also offers benefits beyond diagnostic test numbers, including protection against dementia and cancer, and sustainable weight loss. It improves your overall health and increases your healthy life expectancy. If you are on medication, it is crucial to consult your physician when you embark on this program. It is important that you and your doctor have a plan to gradually lower your medication as your blood pressure improves, so your blood pressure does not become too low and you do not become dangerously overmedicated. This program can lower your blood pressure quickly, and that can place you at risk if your medication is not adjusted accordingly. In most cases, you will be able to eventually discontinue your medication as you lose weight and improve your health.

My approach has been proven to work, and is documented to be the most effective way to lower blood pressure and cholesterol.[1] A study of those following my recommendations, published in *The American Journal of Lifestyle Medicine*, showed dramatic reductions in weight, cholesterol and blood pressure. It also demonstrated the reversal of advanced heart disease. Respondents who were not taking cholesterol-lowering medication experienced an average 42 mg/dl decrease in LDL cholesterol. Those who were hypertensive had a 26 mm Hg average reduction in systolic blood pressure.[1]

I have used this approach with thousands of patients throughout my more than 25 years practicing nutritional medicine. My research has shown that, in most cases, your cholesterol and blood pressure numbers will be lower following this plan than they would be from medication. And when you normalize your blood pressure and cholesterol by earning it through dietary excellence rather than merely covering up the problem with drugs, it is true healing. This approach can save your life.

This program is best utilized in conjunction with the information you will learn in my book, *The End of Heart Disease*. This is a quick guide to immediately get you started while you read and absorb the full details and the science of the entire program in *The End of Heart Disease*. A health transformation is yours to attain in the next 20 days. I hope your results will encourage and motivate you to continue to eat healthfully for the rest of your life.

Wishing you the best of health always,

Joel Fuhrman

TABLE OF CONTENTS

INTRODUCTION

FOOD CAN EITHER KILL OR HEAL.
THE CHOICE IS YOURS.

Let me be crystal clear: Food is the cause of, and should be the solution for, high blood pressure and high cholesterol. Everything else is just window dressing. It is a fact that certain foods lead to superior health and other foods lead to ill health.

A superior diet can restore your health quickly. If you strictly follow the meal plans in this guide, you can significantly lower your blood pressure and cholesterol in less than three weeks. It works.

I know that radically changing your diet can be challenging at first. But once you make the commitment, adapting to a Nutritarian style of eating becomes easy—and can be fun. Strictly following my meal plans will make the adjustment easier, as you reset your palate and learn to savor the flavors of natural food.

This isn't a 20-day diet; rather it is the beginning of a new lifestyle. That's the best part; it's sustainable. Eventually, your sense of taste will get stronger as you get healthier. You will enjoy eating this way more and more—and gradually, unhealthful eating will lose its appeal. Plus, you will lose excess weight in the process. Increasingly, as you learn to prepare and cook healthy foods in creative and tasty ways, you will appreciate that this way of eating is satisfying and delicious. It is a lifestyle—one that you can successfully embrace. It will reset your palate, recharge your mind and re-energize your body as you achieve optimal health.

A Nutritarian lifestyle does more than address one or two heart disease risk factors (unlike taking a cholesterol-lowering medication, or one or more drugs to lower blood pressure). It addresses and repairs scores of conditions governing your future health. For example, the inner lining of the blood vessels becomes smoother and less inflamed, the vessel walls become more elastic, and more oxygenated blood is able to fill the coronary arteries. And critical to your life, your LDL cholesterol is no longer oxidized. It is important to note it is oxidized LDL that is the bad player, because it leads to artery-clogging plaque formation. A Nutritarian diet floods the body with antioxidants that resolve vascular inflammation and radically lower oxidized LDL; you become resistant to heart disease, diabetes and cancer. It also improves your immune function, thereby giving you protection against dangerous infections.

CONNECTIONS

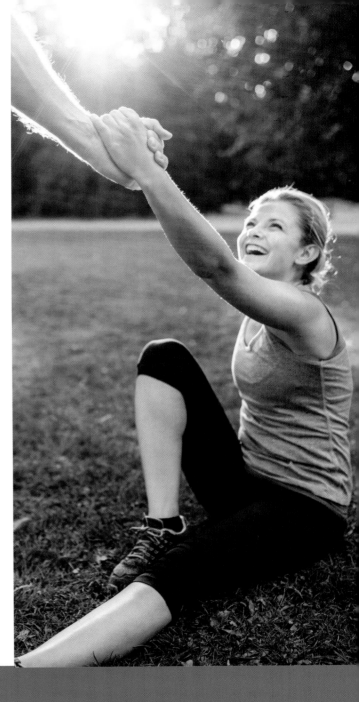

You aren't alone on this journey! An important part of the *Transformation 20 Blood Pressure and Cholesterol* program is being able to connect with those going through the same process. Use this support to keep on track and hold yourself accountable. Get advice, compare notes, and you won't be derailed.

By purchasing this program, you have access to the private Dr. Fuhrman T20 Blood Pressure and Cholesterol Facebook page, where you can interact with others who are following the program. It is a great place to share tips, trade recipes and get inspired!

Join now at
www.facebook.com/groups/DrFuhrmanT20BPC

In addition, membership to DrFuhrman.com will give you access to a wealth of health and nutrition resources, including a Health Tracker so you can monitor your progress, the Nutritarian Recipe Database with over 1,700 recipes, and a dedicated Transformation 20 Blood Pressure and Cholesterol Community where you can post questions. Members also receive generous discounts on Dr. Fuhrman products and have access to our Ask the Doctor Community, plus other exclusive perks.
www.drfuhrman.com/membership

SHOPPING TIP

The ingredients for all of the recipes in this plan are available at your favorite food markets. But it can be a challenge to find prepared foods, such as salad dressings, soups and condiments that are made without added salt, sugar, oils and starches. You'll find these products, as well as multivitamins, supplements, books, and media, at *DrFuhrman.com.*

HIPPOCRATES SAID:
"LET FOOD BE THY MEDICINE"

Studying nutrition's role in health care was a hobby of mine that developed into a passion long before I decided to go to medical school, and it was this passion that drove me to become a physician. Over the years, upon seeing thousands of patients and culling thousands of research articles, I developed an eating style, which has become known as "Nutritarian." It needed its own name as there was no diet style that fit its criteria. It is based on numerous features that promote excellent health and longevity, including my health equation:

$$H = N/C$$

Your health (H) is determined by the nutrients (N) and calories (C) in your diet, also known as the nutrient density of your diet. Here, nutrients mainly refer to the micronutrients in your diet. Micronutrients are vitamins, minerals and phytonutrients (antioxidants). They are the calorie-free nutrients. These micronutrients are key to maintaining a healthy life with an optimal weight.

A Nutritarian diet is one that is rich in the protective nutrients that maximize health and longevity. It includes nutrient-rich, whole plant foods with dramatically fewer animal products, as animal products are devoid of antioxidants and phytonutrients. The diet is rich in vegetables, with an emphasis on greens, but I also recommend the specific inclusion of mushrooms, beans, fruit (especially berries), nuts and seeds, and some intact whole grains. Animal products are permitted, but in much smaller quantities than are usually consumed—they are to be used only in small amounts as a flavoring agent. It is a style of eating that is not only highly effective at preventing disease, but also capable of dramatically reversing chronic diseases, such as type 2 diabetes, heart disease, headaches/migraines, autoimmune diseases, constipation and irritable bowel syndrome.

In addition, it allows you to achieve sustainable weight loss and easily maintain a favorable weight forever, without the need for calorie counting.

By removing low-nutrient processed foods and most animal products from your diet and replacing them with more wholesome, nutrient-rich plant food, you supply your body with an abundance of fiber, essential micronutrients, antioxidants and other phytochemicals necessary for cardiovascular health, cellular repair and optimal immune function. Consuming a large amount of fiber and phytonutrients also lowers cholesterol levels and helps dissolve cholesterol plaque in your arteries.

Cruciferous vegetables, berries, tomatoes and other components of the diet complement the body's natural antioxidant systems to help prevent LDL oxidation, an early step in the process of atherosclerotic plaque formation. Phytochemicals called flavonoids help to restore healthy blood pressure regulation. Also, atherosclerosis is an inflammatory disease, and phytochemicals in green vegetables, berries and other plant foods counteract inflammation. Minimizing added sodium is also crucial to keep blood pressure down and prevent artery walls from stiffening.

In addition to lowering blood pressure and reducing cholesterol, this eating style normalizes body weight by removing from your diet processed foods such as oils, white flour and sweeteners, which promote fat storage on the body.

BENEFITS OF A NUTRITARIAN LIFESTYLE

- Dramatically Lowers Blood Pressure
- Dramatically Reduces Low-Density Lipoprotein (LDL) Cholesterol
- Prevents Oxidation of LDL Cholesterol
- Eliminates Excess Weight
- Resolves Intravascular Inflammation
- Reverses Atherosclerosis (Blood Vessel Plaque)
- Lowers Blood Glucose and Triglyceride Levels
- Improves Exercise Tolerance and Oxygen Efficiency
- Protects Against Heart Disease, Stroke and Other Serious Illnesses
- Slows the Aging Process, Supports Brain Function and Protects Against Dementia

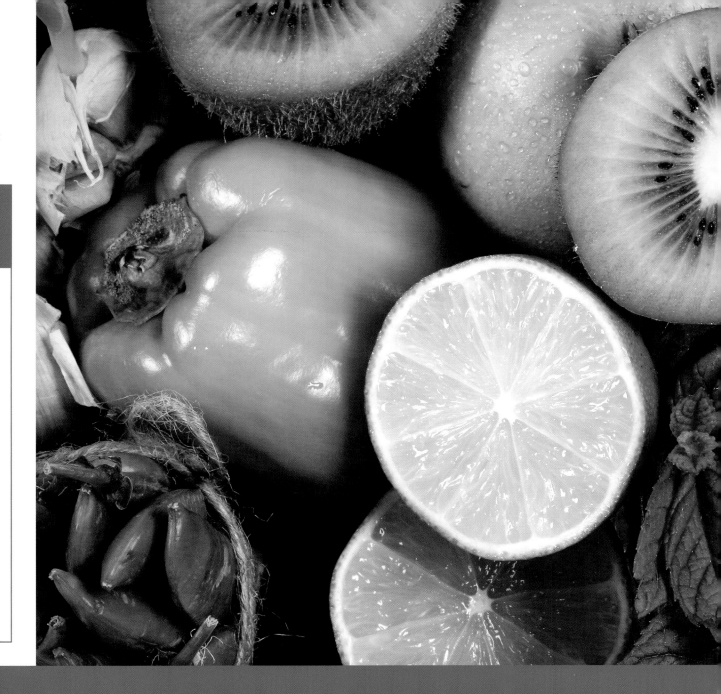

MEDICATIONS ARE NOT THE ANSWER

If you have been diagnosed with high blood pressure or high cholesterol—or both—it is likely that your doctor is treating you with medication, and not putting much emphasis on a change in your diet. But while this conventional, pharmacological approach may help lower your numbers, it does nothing to eliminate the underlying cause of your condition. In addition, medications have their own side effects, some of which are dangerous. Why expose yourself to those risks?

I always say a prescription pad is like a permission slip. You can treat the symptom (elevated blood pressure or cholesterol) with drugs, but that won't prevent the degeneration of your blood vessels, your brain and your heart. These abnormalities will usually continue to advance, in spite of medical care. Then, believing that you are safe with drug-induced normal numbers, you'll think it is acceptable to continue the disease-causing diet that created the problems to begin with. Inevitably, your health will continue to deteriorate, despite the medications. Plus, the medications increase your risk of developing other diseases, such as cancer.

This pharmacological approach hasn't changed the fact that heart disease and strokes are still the leading causes of death for adult Americans. Drugs simply cannot do what a Nutritarian diet can. A program of dietary excellence with appropriate supplementation offers more protection than any medication, since medications don't address what is causing the damage to the blood vessels: the wrong food. In addition, by eating this healthful diet, you will be protecting yourself against a possible heart attack or stroke, and you will also be protecting yourself from other diseases, like cancer and diabetes.

HIGH BLOOD PRESSURE

Hypertension, or high blood pressure, is often called the "silent killer" because it usually does not have clear symptoms. But this condition can quietly cause very serious health problems, such as a kidney insufficiency, deterioration of the brain, strokes, and heart attacks.

Your blood pressure reading consists of two numbers: the first (upper) number is the systolic pressure, which measures the pressure blood exerts against artery walls when the heart contracts. The second (lower) number is the diastolic pressure, which measures the pressure blood exerts when the heart relaxes. Your goal should be to achieve a systolic blood pressure under 125 through nutritional excellence, rather than through medication—because the side effects of blood pressure medications are serious and, in some cases, life-threatening.

Medication to lower systolic blood pressure can lower the diastolic pressure excessively, which can lead to cardiac arrhythmias and—especially in those over the age of 65—can actually increase the risk of heart attack.[2, 3] That is because as blood vessels stiffen with disease and aging, the vessels don't expand as much during systole (which increases pressure), and don't contract as much during diastole. When meds are used to lower the systolic number, this also has the effect of excessively pushing the diastolic number down, potentially to the point where the coronary arteries don't fill adequately during diastole.

You can't take medications without paying a price, due to their toxicity. Diuretics and beta-blockers, two commonly prescribed types of blood pressure meds, have been shown to increase the risk of developing diabetes.[4, 5] Long-term use of diuretics and calcium channel blockers has also been linked to increased incidence of breast cancer.[6, 7]

WHAT IS A **NORMAL** BLOOD PRESSURE?

Blood pressure is expressed as two numbers: the first is systolic pressure, and the second is diastolic pressure. Both numbers represent the pressure the blood exerts against the artery walls. During systole, the heart contracts and sends blood into the arteries and to the rest of the body; systolic pressure is the pressure during systole. During diastole, the heart relaxes and refills.

Normal Blood Pressure
Systolic less than 120 and
Diastolic less than 80

Prehypertension
Systolic 120-139 or
Diastolic 80-89

High Blood Pressure
Hypertension (Stage 1)
Systolic 140-159 or
Diastolic 90-99

High Blood Pressure
Hypertension (Stage 2)
Systolic 160 or higher
or Diastolic 100 or higher

Hypertensive Crisis
Systolic 180 or higher
or Diastolic 110 or higher

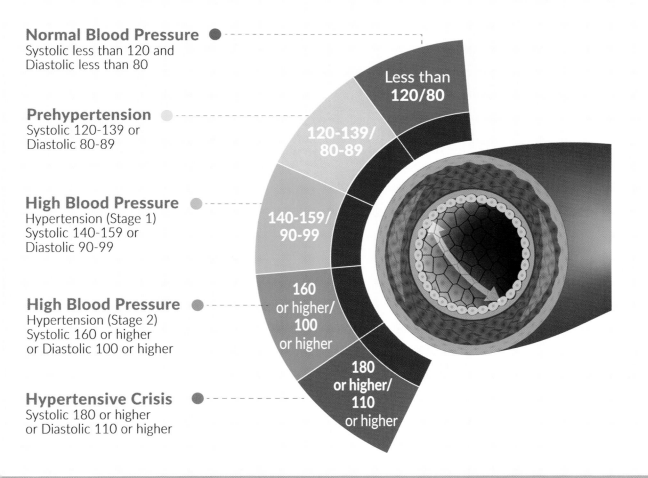

Less than
120/80

120-139/
80-89

140-159/
90-99

160
or higher/
100
or higher

180
or higher/
110
or higher

HIGH CHOLESTEROL

Cholesterol is a type of waxy com
produced in the liver, and is also
the body when we consume anim
animal products provide cholest
not contain any cholesterol. Cholesterol is used
to make steroid hormones and is a component
of cell membranes. We need a certain amount
of cholesterol to survive, and our bodies know
how much to produce on their own. If we eat too
much animal products or processed foods and not
enough high-fiber, high-nutrient foods, we end up
with unhealthy cholesterol levels. LDL is the major
"bad" cholesterol. High levels of small, dense LDL
particles that are oxidized are the most harmful,
promoting plaque buildup in the arteries.

More than a quarter of adults over the age of
45 take statin drugs to lower cholesterol, which
makes this category of medications one of the
most frequently prescribed.[8] But most patients are
unaware that these drugs are associated with serious
side effects, including an elevated risk of type 2
diabetes and kidney injury.[9-11] In addition, there
is controversy over how much protection statin
drug use actually provides, and whether corporate
conflicts of interest have inflated the estimated
reduction in risk of cardiovascular events.[12]

Among the other potential problems associated
with the use of statin drugs are weight gain,
reduced physical fitness, cataracts, myopathies
(muscle damage), sexual dysfunction, fatigue,
memory problems, depression and insomnia. In

...atins inhibit the synthesis of vitamin ...ch is important in preventing coronary ...cations, and deplete stores of coenzyme ...0, a necessary component of cellular energy production.[12]

In contrast, a Nutritarian diet is the safer option. It is more effective at getting rid of the cholesterol inside the atherosclerotic plaque—not just in the blood stream—and it is more effective at inducing disintegration of the plaque. It also eliminates inflammation, and can eventually restore elasticity of our blood vessels. It is more than 100 times as effective at preventing future heart attacks, compared to taking drugs.[13]

It is important to remember that while a diagnosis of high LDL levels is a cause for concern, it is only one of a number of risk factors for heart disease. When you eat healthfully and earn a normal cholesterol and a good blood pressure, the dangerous potential of the LDL particles to form atherosclerotic plaque changes in numerous ways. The high amounts of antioxidants and phytochemicals in the Nutritarian diet transform the size and shape of the LDL molecule and remove oxidized LDL cholesterol, typically making the remaining LDL cholesterol harmless.

Remember: I recommend that medications be slowly reduced with medical supervision as you follow this program. Do not stop them suddenly. Consult your physician before making any changes.

TOTAL CHOLESTEROL
includes various forms of cholesterol, including LDL, HDL and VLDL.

LDL Cholesterol (Low-Density Lipoprotein)

LDL is considered "bad" cholesterol, because elevated LDL makes heart disease more likely to develop. However, it is important to note that it is the oxidized form of LDL that is the bad guy. The oxidized form of LDL travels into arterial walls, where it is modified, taken up by inflammatory cells, and begins to build up as atherosclerotic plaque. This establishes plaque in arteries, which can rupture, creating a clot and causing a heart attack or stroke.

Optimal LDL Level: Less than 100 mg/dl. However, this number misrepresents risk when eating a Nutritarian diet, since this program not only lowers LDL, but prevents oxidation of the LDL. Individuals eating a superior diet—even those with total LDL numbers higher than 100—will be at considerably lower risk due to much of the LDL not being oxidized.

HDL Cholesterol (High-Density Lipoprotein)

HDL is sometimes called a "friendly scavenger" or "good cholesterol," because it moves cholesterol out of the body by carrying it back to the liver for disposal. If your LDL is unfavorable, then a higher HDL is favorable. However, a high HDL level is linked with a lower risk of heart disease only in people eating heart disease-promoting diets. In individuals and populations eating a heart disease-protective diet, a lower HDL is not a disadvantage. The body has no need to produce HDL when there is no unfavorable LDL or cholesterol deposits to remove. So, in people or populations free of heart disease, low HDL levels are common and expected, and not a risk factor. Do not be concerned if, over time, your HDL decreases along with your LDL as you follow this new style of eating.

Optimal HDL Level: Varies based on LDL. May not be a factor with a Nutritarian diet.

VLDL Cholesterol (Very Low-Density Lipoprotein)

VLDL contains small, dense LDL particles that are more atherogenic (capable of producing arterial plaque) than larger LDL particles. High levels of VLDL cholesterol in the blood increase your risk of heart disease and stroke.

Optimal VLDL Level: Less than 30 mg/dl. A Nutritarian diet powerfully lowers VLDL.

THE BEST FOODS
TO LOWER BLOOD PRESSURE AND CHOLESTEROL

To be successful on a Nutritarian diet, you have to be a choosy eater, but not a picky one.

Following this plan may mean adding foods you've never tried before to your regular diet. As adults, we often gravitate to the foods we were raised with, but continuing to eat only familiar foods could be your downfall. Research shows that it takes between eight to fifteen times eating a new food to accept it as familiar. Taste is a learned pattern; it is not fixed. Repeated exposure to a variety of fruits and vegetables

has been shown to increase our acceptance and liking of them.

For superior results, I would like you to accept the notion that, in the beginning, I will choose what you will eat, not you. This makes it easy, because the decision is made for you, and the results will amaze you. With time, your taste preferences will change, and you will learn new recipes that you'll love. Eventually, eating this healthfully will be the way you prefer to eat, and enjoy the most.

THE BEST FOODS

GREEN VEGETABLES

The most nutrient-dense of all foods, green vegetables (especially cruciferous vegetables) contain substances that protect blood vessels, reduce blood pressure, protect against inflammation, and reduce oxidation, the main cause of cardiovascular disease. One way that cruciferous vegetables enhance health is by activating a powerful protein called Nrf2, which stimulates the body's detoxification system and antioxidant enzymes.[14, 15] Greens, especially leafy greens, are also an ideal food for weight control, containing only about 100 calories (but lots of nutrients) per pound.

BEANS

People who eat beans and other legumes regularly take in more minerals and fiber, have lower blood pressure, and are less likely to be overweight than those who don't consume beans.[16] Beans contain soluble fiber, which helps to lower cholesterol.[17] Beans are high in fiber overall, which also is associated with lower blood pressure.[18] Daily consumption of beans helps reduce your appetite and lower your blood sugar. Beans are an ideal weight-loss food because they are digested slowly, promoting satiety.

NUTS AND SEEDS

Nut consumption is consistently associated with a longer life.[19] Both nuts and seeds provide healthy fats, minerals and antioxidants. Seeds have more protein and are abundant in trace minerals. Nuts have anti-inflammatory properties, reduce oxidative stress on cells, lower cholesterol, improve blood vessel function, help with weight maintenance, and lower the glycemic load of meals.[20-22] Daily nut consumption is associated with protection against sudden cardiac death, and enhanced longevity. In an analysis of studies that lasted at least five years, each daily serving of nuts was associated with a 39 percent reduced risk of death from cardiovascular disease, and a 27 percent reduction in risk of death from all causes.[19]

BERRIES

Antioxidant-rich berries help protect against the production of atherosclerotic plaque. They also increase blood antioxidant capacity, decrease adhesion of inflammatory cells to blood vessel walls, and improve blood pressure. Higher berry consumption has been associated with lowering the inflammatory marker C-reactive protein.[23]

POMEGRANATE

This sweet/tart fruit has numerous health benefits. Pomegranates offer punicalagin, a powerful antioxidant unique to that fruit. It, along with the pomegranate's other phytochemicals, have anti-inflammatory and anti-cancer effects. Pomegranate helps to reduce oxidation of (bad) LDL cholesterol (which impedes the build-up of coronary artery plaque) and reduce blood pressure.[24-26]

FLAX

This omega-3-packed seed has lowered systolic and diastolic blood pressure in many clinical studies.[27] It is also a high-fiber food. One or two tablespoons each day is all you need to reap its benefits. Use the seed and not the oil to get the full benefits. Whole flaxseeds need to be ground before eating, and should be stored in the refrigerator or freezer to preserve freshness.

TOMATOES

As the major source of the carotenoid lycopene, a very strong antioxidant, tomatoes (especially cooked tomatoes) are an important food for the cardiovascular system. Lycopene has anti-inflammatory effects and helps LDL to be more resistant to oxidation. A higher level of lycopene in the blood has been linked to a lower risk of heart attack and stroke.[28-32]

ONIONS AND GARLIC

Allium vegetables (like onions and garlic) are effective heart-disease fighters.[33] Garlic has the ability to inhibit cholesterol synthesis, decrease platelet aggregation and prevent oxidation of LDL cholesterol.[34, 35] Onions reduce the risk of cardiovascular disease through their natural anti-clotting abilities and antioxidant compounds.[36, 37] Onions and garlic also possess potent anti-cancer properties.[38, 39]

MUSHROOMS

All types of mushrooms have anti-cancer effects, such as preventing DNA damage, slowing cancer cell growth, and inhibiting angiogenesis. Mushroom phytochemicals have anti-inflammatory effects on endothelial cells, suggesting mushroom intake opposes atherosclerotic plaque development.[40, 41] In a study that assigned participants to either maintain their standard diet, or replace red meat with mushrooms in their meals for one year, the mushroom group lost body fat, and lowered their blood pressure, cholesterol, and C-reactive protein levels.[42] Eat a variety of mushrooms to get all their beneficial properties, but eat them cooked. Raw mushrooms contain a potentially carcinogenic substance called agaritine that is significantly reduced through cooking.[43]

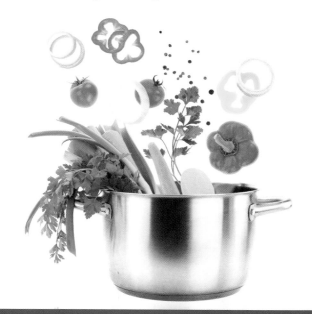

THE WORST FOODS

ADDED SUGARS

Sugar-sweetened beverages and desserts, sugary processed foods, fruit juices, honey, maple and corn syrups, agave nectar and molasses are all low in nutrients and fiber, and cause dangerous elevations in blood glucose (hyperglycemia). Acute hyperglycemia occurring after a meal has been found to promote heart disease by impairing vascular function, suppressing blood flow to the heart, and increasing circulating adhesion molecules.[44-46] Hyperglycemia also results in the production of free radicals and Advanced Glycation End Products (AGEs), which damage body proteins, cause oxidative stress and inflammation, and contribute to blood vessel damage and atherosclerosis.[47, 48]

REFINED GRAINS

Baked goods, cold breakfast cereals, snack foods such as pretzels, white bread, white rice, and white pasta, all lack fiber and other nutrients—and much like added sugars, they elevate blood glucose. A diet containing a lot of these high-glycemic foods promotes insulin resistance, elevated triglycerides, and impaired vascular function, and is associated with a greater risk of heart disease and stroke.[49]

FRIED FOODS

Potato chips, French fries, doughnuts, and other fried starches are high-calorie, low-nutrient foods. Not only do these foods promote weight gain, they are high in AGEs and contain a harmful by-product called acrylamide, because they are cooked at high temperatures.[50-52]

TRANS FATS, MARGARINE AND BUTTER

Trans fats - which were commonly used in margarines and processed foods - dramatically increase cardiovascular risk.53 These dangerous fats (hydrogenated oils) are being phased out in the U.S., but check ingredient labels. Even non-trans-fat margarines and shortening are made of nutrient-depleted oils, and butter increases LDL cholesterol levels.[54].

RED AND PROCESSED MEATS

Overall, eating more animal protein and less plant protein is linked to earlier death.[55-58] Red and processed meat consumption, however, is even more dangerous, associated with the highest rates of heart disease deaths and strokes.[59, 60] The negative cardiovascular effects of red and processed meats are thought to be brought about by a combination of several factors such as heme iron, which promotes oxidation of LDL cholesterol and plaque formation;[61-63] and carnitine and choline, which are converted by gut bacteria to a pro-inflammatory compound that promotes cardiovascular disease.[64, 65]

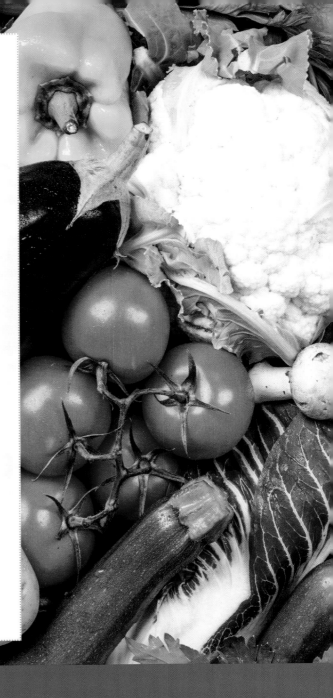

SALT IS A FOUR-LETTER WORD

Salt is dangerous. Whether you use one of the many varieties of sea salt or just the plain kind on the table, they all shorten your life.

Do not add salt to your food, whether or not you have high blood pressure. High salt intake is linked to increases in cardiovascular mortality and serious health problems—in the cardiovascular system and elsewhere—even if blood pressure is not elevated.[66-68] Meaning, even if you have normal blood pressure, salt eventually takes its toll on your health and shortens lifespan. If you don't have high blood pressure and you eat salt, you most likely will develop high blood pressure as you age. But even when your blood pressure remains normal, salt is still damaging your body, creating microvascular hemorrhages and other damage that is cumulative.

Salt also deadens taste buds, desensitizing the palate to more subtle flavors in natural foods. It is an ironic fact that the more salt you use, the flatter the food tastes. As a result, you will desire even more salt in the future.

HIDDEN SALT IN OUR FOOD

Our bodies get an optimal level of sodium from a natural diet, but most Americans consume four to six times what they need. Essential hypertension, the most common category of high blood pressure, is linked to a high-sodium diet. And while it is wise to remove the salt shaker from your dinner table, salt from a salt shaker is not the biggest contributor of sodium in our diet. It only accounts for 11 percent of our salt intake in America. The majority of our salt consumption (77 percent) comes from processed foods, restaurant foods and other prepared foods that are loaded with sodium. Preparing your own food from scratch eliminates the major sources of excess sodium.

The worst offenders are bread, tomato sauces, canned soups, breakfast cereals, condiments and salad dressings. Our standard American diet is loaded with harmful amounts of sodium (and hidden sugars) in processed foods and fast foods.

HOW MUCH IS TOO MUCH SALT?

The average American consumes about 4,000 milligrams of sodium a day.[69] Health authorities such as the American College of Cardiology recommend less than 1,500 mg of sodium per day. My recommendation is to limit your sodium consumption to less than 1,000 milligrams per day. This means less than 400 mg daily of added sodium, since natural foods will give you between 500 and 700 mg per day.

Consuming less salt is among the most important things you can do for your health. A large, long-term study of lifestyle interventions published in 2007 showed that a 25 to 35 percent reduction in dietary sodium over 10 to 15 years resulted in a 25 to 30 percent lower risk of cardiovascular events and cardiovascular deaths.[70]

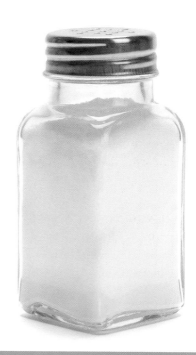

If you just ate natural foods without added salt, you would most likely consume about 500 to 700 milligrams of sodium a day. Even if your blood pressure is low, salting your food may increase your risk of hemorrhagic stroke, kidney stones and kidney malfunction, vascular inflammation, obesity, autoimmune disease, stomach cancer, heart damage and blood vessel damage. In addition, the more salt you eat, the harder it is for your body to hold onto calcium, increasing your probability of osteoporosis (as excess salt is eliminated in the urine, calcium is leached from the body).

FLAVOR FOOD WITHOUT SALT

Not adding salt to your food doesn't mean you must be resigned to a life of bland food. On the contrary, you will be awakening your taste buds to the diversity of natural flavors that you have missed because of salt. (See my suggestions to add flavor without the use of salt.)

After you wean yourself from salt, you will find that your taste preferences change and you will learn to prefer food that is prepared without salt. High blood pressure is not a natural consequence of aging. Mostly, it is a consequence of the sodium in our diet, and excess weight.

NO SALT DOESN'T MEAN NO FLAVOR

Put the salt shaker down and enhance the flavor of your dishes with a splash of lemon, lime or orange juice. Or add a small amount of flavored vinegar for a tang that will awaken your taste buds. In addition to using onions, leeks, shallots, chives, scallions and fresh garlic, try roasting a whole head of garlic in the oven for 25 minutes at 350 degrees F. The softened garlic can be used in dips, spreads and salad dressings for a delicious, buttery flavor. Below are other suggestions to consider when swapping out salt.

GO BIG ON THESE HERBS AND SPICES:

- No-salt seasoning blends like Dr. Fuhrman's VegiZest and MatoZest
- Mrs. Dash
- Nutritional yeast (unfortified)
- Black pepper
- Red pepper flakes
- Cayenne pepper
- Dried chilies
- Chili powder

- Basil
- Cilantro
- Parsley
- Thyme
- Cumin
- Coriander
- Cinnamon
- Vanilla
- Cloves

FREQUENTLY ASKED QUESTIONS

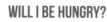 **WILL I BE HUNGRY?**
You will find that your appetite will be more than satisfied from all the nutrients and fiber consumed and over time, as the nutrients in your tissues increase, you will find your cravings gone and you will lose the drive to eat too frequently and too much. The fiber, plant protein and fats in beans, vegetables, nuts and seeds provide the same feelings of fullness and satiety as the protein and fat in unhealthy foods, but in a health-promoting package. You will be able to eat a large, filling amount of food while consuming a small amount of calories, and feel no hunger or deprivation.

 WILL I EXPERIENCE ANY DISCOMFORT FROM SWITCHING TO SUCH A HEALTHY DIET?
As detoxification from your former diet begins, you may feel some lightheadedness, fatigue, headaches, shakiness and irritability. I call these uncomfortable feelings 'toxic hunger,' and they usually occur a few hours after eating. The good news is that toxic hunger usually disappears within a few days of starting a high-nutrient diet. It is a lot like going through withdrawal after quitting caffeine. You may also experience some bloating or gas as your body adjusts to the increase in fiber. Chewing your food thoroughly will help.

HOW DO I EAT AT A RESTAURANT ON THIS PLAN?
Dining out may seem challenging at first. However, taking just a little time to plan ahead makes it much easier. Many more health-oriented eating establishments are opening across the country. Check the menus of

local restaurants online, and find a few that have healthful options. Oatmeal and fresh fruit are easy to find for breakfast. For either lunch or dinner, your best bet is a large, entree-size salad, either with dressing on the side (use only a small amount) or lemon juice or vinegar instead of dressing. Add beans, tofu or Portobello mushrooms if they have those options to make it more filling. Another good option is to request a meal out of a few of the vegetable side dishes on the menu. Make sure to ask for your vegetables without salt or oil. With a little time, you will get to know the restaurants in your area that will accommodate your dietary needs, and you'll get better at scanning menus for healthful options.

IS THIS PLAN ALL OR NOTHING? WILL I GET ANY BENEFIT IF I EAT THIS WAY HALF OF THE TIME?

The benefits you get out of this plan will be proportional to the effort you put in. In my more than 25 years of experience with patients, I have observed that when they go all the way and make a full commitment, it is so much easier, and the results are spectacular. By committing to follow the plan 100 percent instead of 80 or 90 percent, you avoid the constant stress of decision-making. You never have to make a difficult choice in the moment if you have already decided to eat only healthful foods.

HOW CAN I DO THIS PLAN IF I DON'T HAVE ENOUGH TIME TO COOK?

The idea of fitting hours of food preparation into an already busy life may feel overwhelming. But it doesn't have to take much time. Nutritarian meals can range from quick and easy to complex, gourmet cuisine. My *Eat to Live Quick and Easy Cookbook* is a great resource for fast, easy recipes. I've also included some great tasting recipes here, and you can find more online as a member of *DrFuhrman.com*. An example for an on-the-go lunch: raw vegetables dipped in low-salt hummus, followed by a piece of fruit. As long as you keep your kitchen stocked, you can make a great salad in just a few minutes. Mix prewashed mixed greens with shredded cabbage and carrots (or pre-packaged broccoli slaw), canned beans, and chopped walnuts. Top with nut butter mashed with flavored vinegar or lemon juice, and you're ready to eat. Finish with a piece of fruit, or cut up some fruit and add it to the salad.

I have also produced some salad dressings, sauces and soups to make sure even the busiest people can recover their health. So even if you have no time, there are no excuses. You can get out of danger and earn good health.

IS IT TRUE THAT RED WINE IS HEART-HEALTHY?

Red wine does contain some flavonoids and the antioxidant resveratrol. However, adding red wine to an already healthful, high-antioxidant diet likely will not provide any additional benefits, and actually could be detrimental to your health. Even light drinking is associated with an increased risk of cancer.[71]

The anti-clotting benefits that have been observed with moderate red wine drinking are only favorable for people who are eating the unhealthful standard American diet. Alcohol interferes with blood clotting, so only those who have an abnormally high risk of clotting (from eating unhealthfully) would benefit from this action.[72] The blood thinning effects from regular alcohol consumption can increase risk of hemorrhagic stroke.

WHAT ABOUT OLIVE OIL FOR HEART HEALTH? IS A NUTRITARIAN DIET BETTER THAN A MEDITERRANEAN DIET?

A Mediterranean diet is only a small step up from the standard American diet, and most deaths in Mediterranean countries still come from heart disease and strokes, so it is far from optimal. Similarly, olive oil is better than butter and animal fat, but it is still fattening; whereas eating whole foods instead, such as nuts, seeds, and avocado, have proven benefits to lower heart attack risk. Unlike oil, nuts and seeds contain fiber that both slows the absorption of calories, and, importantly, binds cholesterol and removes it from the body. Oils provide lots of calories and no fiber, which promotes weight gain, whereas nuts have been found to help maintain a healthy weight.[73]

The traditional Mediterranean diet is better than the standard American diet because it includes an abundance of health-promoting unrefined plant foods, like vegetables, fruits, nuts, beans and grains, but it includes other health-depleting foods, like white flour, salt and oil.

A Nutritarian diet contains all of the healthy characteristics of a Mediterranean diet, and adds more. It avoids white flour, salt and oil, reduces dairy and meats, and emphasizes the daily consumption of cruciferous vegetables, berries and beans over grains. It is a portfolio of inclusions and exclusions that maximize human lifespan.

WHY ARE LEAN ANIMAL FOODS LIKE CHICKEN AND FAT-FREE MILK MINIMIZED?

Lean animal foods, like chicken and fat-free milk, contain high amounts of animal protein. Diets high in animal protein are linked to a greater risk of heart disease, cancer and premature death.[58, 74, 75] Decades ago, total fat was thought to be the major dietary factor we should reduce to lessen the risk of heart disease. Unfortunately, this resulted in the misconception that lower-fat animal products and refined carbohydrates are healthy choices. They are not. High animal protein foods are risky, especially when it comes to cancer.[76, 77] Other components of animal foods, such as carnitine, promote inflammation and cardiovascular disease.[64, 65] Excess heme iron from animal foods is also a problem as we get older, because it promotes oxidation of LDL cholesterol and a rise in blood pressure, leading to an increased risk of heart disease and stroke.[60, 62, 63, 78] Overall, the goal is to eat more whole plant foods and fewer animal foods, and processed foods.

I'VE HEARD THAT SATURATED FAT ISN'T THE REAL CULPRIT IN HEART DISEASE, SUGAR IS. DO I STILL NEED TO AVOID BUTTER, RED MEAT AND CHEESE?

Saturated fat is a controversial and misunderstood topic. Every fat-containing food contains some combination of saturated, monounsaturated and polyunsaturated fats. Increasing saturated fat intake has been shown to increase LDL cholesterol levels.[15]

However, when you compare low saturated-fat intake to high saturated-fat intake, often you don't see a difference in heart disease risk, because low saturated-fat intake in most of these studies indicates high refined carbohydrate intake— people avoiding red meat, cheese and butter, but eating lots of white rice, bread, pasta and sugar. That's the problem: If you eat a lesser amount of saturated fat-rich foods, you must eat something else instead. The problem with a lot of the studies is that the people with low saturated-fat intake were making up the loss of saturated-fat calories with calories from unrefined carbohydrates, like pasta, white rice, bread and sugar. It's not that saturated fat isn't harmful—it's that refined carbohydrate is just as bad. When the research has taken into account what people are eating instead of saturated fat, those studies show that replacing saturated fat-rich foods with polyunsaturated fat-rich foods (like nuts and seeds) or high-fiber carbohydrate foods (like beans and intact whole grains), risk is reduced.[16-18] More nuts and beans and less meat and dairy (and refined carbohydrate) is better for heart health.

The bottom line: Saturated fat-rich animal foods and refined carbohydrate foods are both bad for heart health. It's not one or the other.

SHOULD I EAT FISH FOR THE OMEGA-3S?

Omega-3 DHA and EPA are crucial for brain health, and it is imperative to maintain adequate levels of these fatty acids.[79-82] Many people eat fish as their primary source of these omega-3s, but fish is not a favorable source of EPA and DHA. Other than the valuable DHA and EPA, fish does not provide any additional health benefit. It adds animal protein, is not rich in micronutrients like beans and nuts, and importantly, often contains high levels of pollutants such as methylmercury and PCBs. Wild salmon does contain lower levels of PCBs than farmed, so if you do eat salmon or other seafood occasionally, wild is the better choice.[83]

My opinion is that the benefits of eating fish do not outweigh the risks—especially when you can get all the benefits and none of the risks from an algae-based omega-3 supplement. Additionally, an algae-based DHA and EPA, such as my DHA+EPA Purity, is a more sustainable option, and it is free of the environmental pollutants that accumulate in the fatty tissues of fish. If you do eat fish, I recommend limiting your consumption to 6 ounces per week, and sticking with varieties that are lowest in mercury, such as trout, flounder, oysters, sardines, shrimp, pollock and wild salmon.[84]

IMPORTANT SUPPLEMENTS

I recommend that everyone take a safe multivitamin and mineral supplement (or the individual nutrients listed below), plus the omega-3 fatty acids DHA and EPA. Additional supplements may be useful for people with elevated blood pressure or cholesterol. More information can be found on my Vitamin Advisor at DrFuhrman.com/vitamin-advisor.

CHOOSING A MULTIVITAMIN

Even the most healthful diet will leave some nutritional gaps, and I recommend using a carefully designed multivitamin and mineral supplement to optimize your intake of essential vitamins and minerals. The following are the important ingredients to look for in a multi:

VITAMIN B12: Plant foods do not contain vitamin B12, and absorption of B12 becomes less efficient as we age. Vitamin B12 contributes to brain function, red blood cell production and DNA synthesis. Additionally, adequate B12 levels also benefit cardiovascular health by preventing elevation of homocysteine; high homocysteine is linked to heart disease and stroke.[85]

VITAMIN D: Sun exposure is most people's primary source of vitamin D, but may not be enough all year round. Also, too much sun exposure damages the skin. Adequate vitamin D suppresses inflammation, helps to keep blood pressure down, and prevents atherosclerotic plaque development.[86] Low vitamin D levels are very common, and are linked to osteoporosis, depression, autoimmune disease, cancer and diabetes.[87] I recommend supplementing to keep blood levels between 30 and 45 ng/ml.

VITAMIN K2: A Nutritarian diet supplies abundant vitamin K1 in green vegetables, but plant foods are low in vitamin K2. I recommend taking supplemental K2 for bone and cardiovascular health. In the cardiovascular system, vitamin K2 helps to maintain elasticity of the artery wall and prevent stiffening and calcification.[88-90]

IODINE: The body needs iodine to synthesize thyroid hormones, and the primary iodine source for most Americans is iodized salt. Since the Nutritarian diet is low in added salt, I recommend taking supplemental iodine.[91]

ZINC: The zinc in plant foods is less absorbable than zinc in animal foods. The immune system needs adequate zinc, and zinc also supports hundreds of different chemical reactions.[92, 93]

AVOID MULTIVITAMINS WITH THESE INGREDIENTS

Some nutrients may be harmful in supplement form. When shopping for a multivitamin, don't choose one that includes these nutrients:[94-98]

- Beta-carotene
- Vitamin A
- Vitamin E
- Folic acid
- Copper

POTENTIALLY HELPFUL SUPPLEMENTS FOR ELEVATED BLOOD PRESSURE OR CHOLESTEROL

OMEGA-3 DHA AND EPA

The long-chain omega-3 fatty acids DHA and EPA help to maintain brain health throughout all stages of life.[99] Omega-3 supplementation has been shown to improve triglyceride levels, and adequate blood levels are linked to lower risk of heart disease.[100-102] A 2017 meta-analysis of randomized controlled trials of DHA-EPA supplementation determined that DHA-EPA supplementation reduced the risk of coronary heart disease by approximately 15 percent in people with elevated LDL or triglycerides.[103] DHA and EPA may also help to prevent arrhythmias, and their anti-inflammatory effects may inhibit atherosclerosis. As with many nutrients, more is not necessarily better, and high-dose supplements may do more harm than good.[104] I recommend supplementing with about 250 mg/day DHA and EPA from an algae-derived source—because the algae is grown in a lab, there are no pollutants and it is more sustainable than fish oil.

PLANT STEROLS (PHYTOSTEROLS)

Plant sterols occur naturally in nuts, soybeans and other plant foods, and plant sterol supplements have been extensively researched and shown to be effective at lowering LDL cholesterol.[105] When we consume plant sterols, they block the absorption of cholesterol from food and the reabsorption of cholesterol produced by the liver, resulting in lower blood cholesterol levels.

GREEN TEA EXTRACT

Drinking green tea regularly is associated with a reduced risk of heart disease, a ten percent lower risk for each cup of green tea per day.[106] Randomized controlled trials have been conducted to test whether extracts of green tea, prepared as supplements, could improve cardiovascular risk factors. The results so far have been encouraging—green tea extracts have been found to reduce total cholesterol and LDL cholesterol and systolic blood pressure.[107]

CURCUMIN

Curcumin, a combination of phytochemicals from the turmeric root, is known for its anti-inflammatory effects. Chronic inflammation, primarily due to a poor diet and sedentary lifestyle, is one of the root causes of cardiovascular disease. Reductions in circulating C-reactive protein (a marker of chronic inflammation and risk factor for cardiovascular disease) have been observed following curcumin supplementation.[108, 109]

> For additional information regarding the health benefits of Dr. Fuhrman's multivitamins and supplements, please visit the **Vitamin Advisor** at
> **www.DrFuhrman.com/vitamin-advisor**

THE
GROUND RULES

BEFORE YOU GET STARTED . . .

You can anticipate that your blood pressure, cholesterol and blood sugar numbers will fall with this diet and lifestyle plan. If you are taking any medication, especially medication for high blood pressure or diabetes, stay in close communication with your physician, as your medication will need adjustment to prevent excessive lowering of your blood pressure and blood sugar levels.

The menus can be adjusted to meet your caloric needs. They provide about 1,400 calories per day, but you don't need to eat all the food listed if you don't require that many calories. For maximal results you should eat only when hungry; never eat until you are uncomfortable, and don't overeat. For most people, eating sensible amounts of these supplied menus will result in favorable weight loss. But, depending on your age, sex, weight and physical activity level, you may have gradual weight loss, or these menus may be the right amount for weight maintenance. If you have higher calorie requirements and do not wish to lose weight, increase the portion sizes of the menu items. Do not increase portion sizes of animal products.

If you are a bit hungry, but still want to maximize results and maintain weight loss, you can eat more of the lower-calorie, "eat liberally" foods such as raw vegetables, cooked green and non-starchy vegetables and beans at mealtime.

However, it is important to recognize that you shouldn't overeat any food. Try very hard not to eat any food between meals—even if it is listed in the "eat liberally" section. You should feel hungry before eating a meal; this helps ensure that you are not chronically overeating. If you are not hungry at dinnertime, then you likely overate at lunch. If you are not hungry for lunch, you likely overate at breakfast.

Refer to the next page for the chart of Foods to Eat Liberally, Eat in Moderation or Avoid Entirely

The *Transformation 20 Blood Pressure and Cholesterol* program is based on eating large quantities of raw and cooked vegetables. These foods fill you up and leave little room for processed, refined foods, which contain lots of calories but few nutrients. Nutrient-dense vegetables are the most important foods to focus on for disease prevention and reversal. Aim for between a half pound to a full pound of raw vegetables and the same amount of cooked vegetables each day. To give you a general idea, a pound of raw vegetables is a salad composed of 5 cups of chopped romaine lettuce, 1 cup of shredded cabbage, 1 medium tomato, 1 small carrot and ¼ cup chopped raw onion. For cooked portions, 1 ½ cups of broccoli is about 8 ounces and 1 ½ cups of kale weighs 7 ounces.

Lunch and dinner recipes are interchangeable, so feel free to swap meals within these categories or repeat a meal more often than it is on the menu. When you have leftovers, they can be substituted for other meals. If you like a recipe, double it and freeze it in individual portions so you don't have to do as much cooking. Just don't have a meal that contains bread more than three times a week, and don't have a breakfast meal more than once a day. Limit animal products to 6 ounces or less per week.

Frozen vegetables and fruit can be substituted for fresh. Don't use canned vegetables or fruit. Canned products lose nutrients during processing and often contain added sugar or salt. Choose products that are no-salt-added or low sodium, and do not add salt to the recipes.

As you change your diet and stop eating unhealthy, addictive foods, your body may go through a detox or withdrawal phase during which you feel weak or uncomfortable, or experience headaches, or have cravings for certain foods. This means that your body is removing toxins and healing. These symptoms will start to resolve gradually as you flood your body with high-nutrient, whole plant foods. The discomfort rarely continues after the first week.

Chew your food very well, until it feels liquefied in your mouth before swallowing. It takes the digestive tract time to adjust to a high-fiber diet that contains lots of raw vegetables and beans. Chewing well will help ease the digestive process and also ensures that more nutrients are available for absorption.

FOODS TO EAT LIBERALLY,
EAT IN MODERATION, OR AVOID ENTIRELY

Whether you want to lose weight or just eat more healthfully, an easy way to make the right dietary choices is to sort foods into three categories: eat liberally, eat in moderation or avoid entirely. The term "eat liberally" is more accurate than the term "unlimited." Unlimited could imply overeating or recreational or emotional eating when not hungry. Also, consuming too much of a very healthy food such as fruit can lead to insufficient vegetables in your diet.

FOLLOW THESE GUIDELINES:

EAT LIBERALLY

You can eat as much as you want of these foods (within reason):

- **Raw vegetables** *(Goal: about ½ to 1 pound daily)*
- **Cooked green and non-green nutrient-dense vegetables** *(Goal: about ½ to 1 pound daily)* Non-green nutrient-dense veggies are: tomatoes, cauliflower, eggplant, mushrooms, peppers, onions and carrots
- **Beans, legumes, lentils, tempeh and edamame** *(Goal: ½-1 cup daily)*
- **Fresh or frozen fruit** *(Goal: 3-5 per day)*

LIMITED *(Eat in Moderation)*

Include these foods in your diet, but limit the amount you are eating:

- **Cooked starchy vegetables or whole grains** *(Maximum: 2 servings daily; 1 serving = 1 cup or 1 slice)*
  - Butternut and other winter squashes
  - Sweet potatoes *(avoid white potatoes)*
  - Corn
  - Quinoa, farro, wild rice or other intact whole grains
  - 100 percent whole grain bread
- **Raw nuts and seeds.** Half should be walnuts or chia, hemp, or flax seeds *(Eat at least 1 ounce or ¼ cup per day; if you are overweight, limit to a maximum of 2 ounces for women or 3 ounces for men)*
- **Avocado** *(Maximum ½ per day)*
- **Dried Fruit** *(Maximum 2 tablespoons per day)*
- **Animal Products: fat-free dairy, clean wild fish and certified organic poultry** *(Maximum of 6 ounces per week, best to limit serving size to 2 ounces, used as a condiment)*

Note: Amounts of cooked starchy vegetables, intact whole grains, nuts, seeds and avocado may be moderately increased depending on your caloric needs.

OFF-LIMITS *(Avoid Entirely)*

- **Products made with sugar, honey, maple syrup or white flour**
- **Soda and soft drinks** including those made with artificial sweeteners
- **Fruit Juice**
- **Barbecued, processed and cured meats, and all red meat**
- **Full-fat and reduced-fat dairy** *(cheese, ice cream, butter, milk)*
- **Eggs**
- **All vegetable oils, including olive oil and coconut oil**

Note: If you are not trying to lose weight, a small amount of olive oil, a teaspoon a day or less, may be used.

STOCK YOUR PANTRY

Before you begin the meal plan, clean out your refrigerator and cabinets of all trigger foods or designate a space for your healthy foods. Stock your pantry with these staple items. They will be needed for the recipes and meals you will be preparing for the next 20 days. Four additional shopping lists are also included with the menus. These are compiled for five-day periods and include perishable items and other foods specific to each set of menus.

NUTS AND SEEDS

All nuts and seeds should be raw and unsalted

Walnuts

Cashews

Almonds

Chia seeds

Hemp seeds

Flax seeds

Sesame seeds

Pumpkin seeds

Sunflower seeds

Raw almond butter

Natural no-salt-added peanut butter

WHOLE GRAINS, DRIED FRUIT, VINEGARS AND OTHER ITEMS

Old-fashioned rolled oats and steel-cut oats

100 percent whole-grain flour tortillas, such as Ezekiel or Alvarado Street brands (store in freezer)

100 percent whole-grain pitas, such as Ezekiel or Alvarado Street brands (store in freezer)

Rice vinegar

Apple cider vinegar

Balsamic vinegar

Fruit-flavored vinegar

Bragg Liquid Aminos or low-sodium soy sauce

Nutritional yeast

Dijon mustard

Dates

Raisins

Unsweetened dried shredded coconut

Wild rice

Quinoa

Farro

Natural non-alkalized cocoa powder

Arrowroot powder

DRIED HERBS AND SPICES

No-salt seasoning blend such as Dr. Fuhrman's VegiZest or Mrs. Dash

No-salt seasoning blend such as Dr. Fuhrman's MatoZest or Italian seasoning blend

Garlic powder

Onion powder

Black pepper

Dried oregano

Dried basil

Coriander

Cumin

Chili powder

Curry powder

Paprika

Thyme

Rosemary

Turmeric

Crushed red pepper flakes

Cinnamon

Alcohol-free vanilla extract

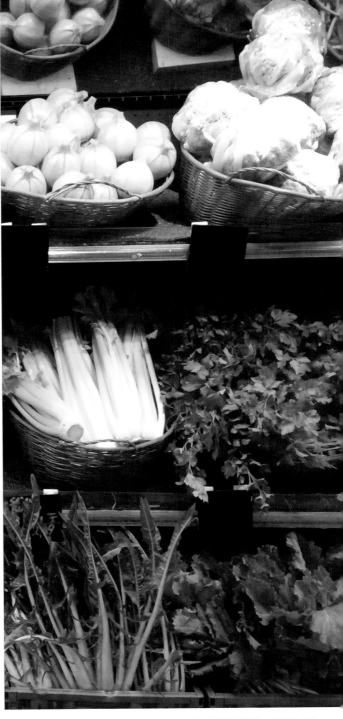

DAYS 1-5
SHOPPING LIST

This shopping list assumes that all recipes in the meal plan will be made. Menus frequently include fruit for dessert and will mention a specific fruit as an example. That fruit is used for the shopping list.

Make sure you also have all the items listed in the Stock Your Pantry list.

FRESH PRODUCE

VEGETABLES

- [ ] 3 heads romaine lettuce
- [ ] 10 ounces mixed baby greens (10 cups)
- [ ] 2 heads of Boston or 1 head of green leaf lettuce (about 10 cups)
- [ ] 3 bunches kale
- [ ] 10 ounces spinach (5 ounces may be frozen)
- [ ] 1 small red cabbage
- [ ] 1 head broccoli (about 7 cups of florets)
- [ ] 1 bunch asparagus
- [ ] 7 ounces green beans (could also buy frozen)
- [ ] Your choice of a green vegetable equal to 2 cups cooked (could also buy frozen)
- [ ] 1 red or green bell pepper
- [ ] 1 jalapeno pepper
- [ ] 2 cucumbers
- [ ] Carrots

- [ ] Celery
- [ ] 4 tomatoes
- [ ] 4 plum tomatoes
- [ ] 2 pounds zucchini (about 5 medium)
- [ ] 2 pounds white or cremini mushrooms
- [ ] 1 avocado
- [ ] 2 medium red or golden beets
- [ ] 7 yellow onions
- [ ] 2 red onions
- [ ] Scallions
- [ ] 2 bulbs garlic
- [ ] Ginger root
- [ ] Parsley
- [ ] Basil

FRUIT

- [ ] 4 ½ cups blueberries (3 cups could be frozen)
- [ ] ½ pound organic strawberries (could use frozen which do not need to be organic)
- [ ] 2 oranges
- [ ] 1 bunch grapes
- [ ] 1 melon, any variety
- [ ] 2 apples (one should be Granny Smith)
- [ ] 2 ½ cups pineapple chunks (could also use frozen)
- [ ] 7 bananas
- [ ] 1 lemon
- [ ] 2 limes

REFRIGERATED

- [ ] 3 cups unsweetened, unflavored soy, hemp or almond milk
- [ ] 2 (14 ounce) packages firm tofu (8 ounces of cooked chicken or shrimp can be substituted for 1 package)

FROZEN

This list does not include vegetables and fruit listed under fresh produce that have a frozen option.

- [ ] Corn kernels (need 2 cups)
- [ ] Strawberries (need 6)
- [ ] Mango (need ½ cup)

SHELF STABLE

BEANS

It is assumed that except for the lentils, canned beans will be used. Select no-salt-added varieties. If you opt to start with dry beans, 1 cup of dry beans will yield about 3 cups of cooked beans

- [ ] 1 (15 ounce) can black beans
- [ ] 2 (15 ounce) cans red beans
- [ ] 2 (15 ounce) cans chick peas
- [ ] 3 (15 ounce) cans white beans
- [ ] 1 cup dried lentils

OTHER

Choose tomato products packaged in BPA-free materials.

- [ ] 5 (32 ounce) cartons no-salt-added vegetable broth
- [ ] Low-sodium salsa (need about 2 cups) If you choose to make your own, add the ingredients in the Day 1 Lunch salsa recipe to your shopping list.
- [ ] No-salt-added diced tomatoes (need 1 ½ cups)
- [ ] No-salt-added tomato paste (need 1/3 cup)
- [ ] No-salt-added tomato sauce (need 1/3 cup)
- [ ] Coconut water (need 1 cup)
- [ ] Caraway seeds
- [ ] Garam masala (an Indian spice blend) or you could use curry powder.
- [ ] Almond extract

DAY 1

Your health is in your hands—primarily the one that holds your fork.

BREAKFAST

BANANA WALNUT BREAKFAST
1 SERVING

1 banana
1 tablespoon ground flax seeds
1 cup blueberries or other berries
¼ cup walnut pieces
¾ cup unsweetened soy, hemp or almond milk

Slice banana into a cereal bowl. Stir in flax seeds, blueberries, walnut pieces, and non-dairy milk.

LUNCH

BLACK BEAN AND AVOCADO SALAD WITH MIXED GREENS
1 SERVING

1 cup cooked or no-salt-added canned black beans, drained
1 tablespoon lime juice
2 tablespoons chopped red onion
¼ teaspoon ground cumin
black pepper, to taste
½ avocado, peeled and diced
5 cups mixed greens
¼ cup no-salt-added salsa (see note)

Combine the beans, lime juice, onion, cumin and black pepper. Gently mix in the avocado. Serve on a bed of mixed greens, topped with the salsa.

Note: To make your own salsa, mix together 2 chopped tomatoes, 1 small chopped red onion, 1 clove minced garlic, ½ chopped jalapeño, 3 tablespoons cilantro and 3 tablespoons lime juice.

Steamed broccoli or other fresh or frozen green vegetable

Orange or other fruit for dessert

> **Tip:** Feel free to adjust the herbs and spices in any of the recipes to suit your preferences. Just don't add salt.

DINNER

CREAMY ZUCCHINI AND CORN SOUP
3 SERVINGS

1 large onion, chopped
3 cloves garlic, chopped
2 pounds zucchini (about 5 medium), chopped
1 teaspoon dried basil
½ teaspoon dried thyme
½ teaspoon dried oregano
4 cups no-salt-added vegetable broth
¼ cup raw cashews or ⅛ cup raw cashew butter
2 tablespoons hemp seeds
4 cups spinach
2 cups frozen corn kernels
¼ teaspoon black pepper or to taste

Add onion, garlic, zucchini, basil, thyme, oregano and vegetable broth to a large soup pot. Bring to a boil, reduce heat and simmer for 25 minutes or until zucchini is tender.

Pour into a high-powered blender (in batches, if necessary), add the cashews and hemp seeds and blend until smooth and creamy.

Return soup to the pot, add corn and spinach, bring to a simmer and cook until spinach is wilted. Add water if needed to adjust consistency. Season with black pepper.

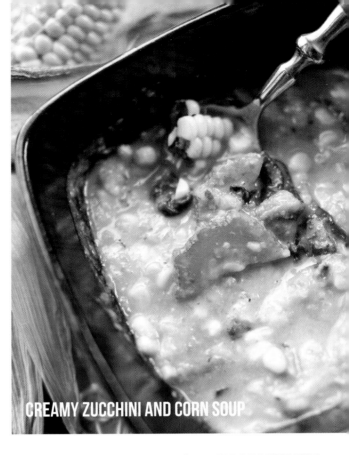

CREAMY ZUCCHINI AND CORN SOUP

MIXED GREEN SALAD WITH CURRIED PEANUT BUTTER DRESSING

Include romaine lettuce, baby greens, tomatoes and red onion in your salad

To make Curried Peanut Butter Dressing, whisk together 2 tablespoons natural peanut butter, 1 teaspoon curry powder, ½ teaspoon Bragg Liquid Aminos, 1 teaspoon lime juice, 2 teaspoons rice vinegar and 3 tablespoons warm water. Add more water if needed to adjust consistency.

Grapes or other fruit for dessert

> **Tip:** Leftovers can be enjoyed as an alternative lunch or dinner. Refrigerate and use within 3-4 days or portion into individual containers and freeze for later use. (See Ground Rules on page 18).

DAY 2

The decision is yours: Choose a favorable diet-style and lifestyle that can effectively protect your health, or rely on drugs and surgical procedures which cannot.

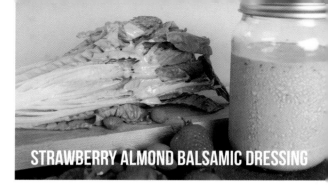

STRAWBERRY ALMOND BALSAMIC DRESSING

BREAKFAST

BLUEBERRY CHIA SOAKED OATS
1 SERVING

½ cup uncooked old-fashioned oats
1 tablespoon chia seeds
1 cup unsweetened soy, hemp or almond milk
2 tablespoons currants or raisins
½-1 cup fresh or thawed frozen blueberries (or other berries)
2 tablespoons chopped raw almonds

Combine the oats, chia seeds, non-dairy milk and raisins. Soak for at least 30 minutes or overnight.

Stir in blueberries and almonds.

LUNCH

Big Green Salad with Strawberry Balsamic Dressing

Include romaine, shredded red cabbage, tomatoes, chopped scallions and ½ cup chickpeas in your salad.

> **Tip:** When it comes to salads, think really big! Include at least 5 cups of leafy lettuce greens.

STRAWBERRY ALMOND BALSAMIC DRESSING
4 SERVINGS

½ pound fresh organic strawberries (hulled) or frozen strawberries
½ cup raw almonds or ¼ cup raw almond butter
2 tablespoons balsamic vinegar
1 teaspoon almond extract

1 tablespoon raisins

Blend all ingredients in a high-powered blender until creamy. Add a few tablespoons of water, if needed, to reach desired consistency.

If you have leftover dressing, you can use it on your salad at lunch on Day 3 or 4.

Steamed asparagus or other green vegetable
(or leftover Zucchini and Corn Soup from Day 1)

Melon or other fruit for dessert

DINNER

LEMONY MUSHROOM QUINOA
3 SERVINGS

1 cup quinoa, rinsed
2 cups no-salt-added vegetable broth
1 pound mushrooms, chopped
2 cloves garlic, chopped
4 scallions, white and light green parts, sliced
¼ cup chopped fresh parsley
1 fresh lemon, juiced and zested
2 tablespoons balsamic vinegar
¼ cup chopped walnuts
½ teaspoon ground black pepper or to taste

Combine quinoa and vegetable stock and cook for 15 minutes or until quinoa is tender. While quinoa is cooking, place mushrooms in a sauté pan over medium heat. When mushrooms begin to give off juice, add garlic and continue to cook for 1-2 minutes.

Combine quinoa, mushrooms and remaining ingredients in large bowl and gently combine. Serve at room temperature.

PERFECT KALE SAUTÉ
2 SERVINGS

1 small onion, thinly sliced
1 clove garlic, chopped
¼ teaspoon crushed red pepper flakes or to taste
1 bunch kale, leaves removed from tough stems and chopped

In a large pan, water sauté onion, garlic and red pepper flakes until the onions start to soften. Add half of the kale, stir for 1 minute then add the remaining kale. Add additional water, as needed, to prevent sticking. Continue cooking 2-4 minutes or until kale is tender.

> **Tip:** Menus can be adjusted to meet your caloric needs. (See Ground Rules on page 18)

HEALTHY MOOSE TRACKS ICE CREAM
2 SERVINGS

1 ripe banana, frozen
½ teaspoon alcohol-free vanilla extract or pure vanilla bean powder
1 tablespoon natural cocoa powder
⅓ cup unsweetened hemp, soy or almond milk
6 frozen strawberries
2 regular or 1 Medjool date, pitted
1 tablespoon ground flax seed
1 tablespoon raw almond butter

Blend all ingredients in a high-powered blender.

Freeze the other serving and enjoy it for dessert tomorrow.

DAY 3

Side effects of the Nutritarian diet include improving your overall health, feeling more energetic and losing weight effortlessly.

BREAKFAST

ISLAND BREEZE SMOOTHIE
1 SERVING

1 cup coconut water
½ ripe banana
½ cup frozen mango chunks
½ cup fresh or frozen pineapple chunks
2 cups chopped kale
½ inch piece fresh ginger

Add ingredients to a high-powered blender and blend until smooth.

LUNCH

Raw Veggies or Green Salad with leftover Curried Peanut Butter Dressing from Day 1 or Strawberry Almond Balsamic from Day 2

SEASONED LENTILS WITH SPINACH
3 SERVINGS

1 onion, chopped
2 stalks celery, chopped
2 carrots, chopped
3 cloves garlic, crushed
1 teaspoon garam masala
1 teaspoon cumin
1 tablespoon minced fresh rosemary or 1 teaspoon dried
3 cups no-salt-added vegetable broth

1 cup dried lentils, rinsed
5 ounces fresh or thawed frozen spinach

In a large soup pot, heat 2-3 tablespoons water and water sauté the onions, celery, carrots and garlic until the carrots are tender and the onion is translucent. Add remaining ingredients except for the spinach and bring to a boil. Reduce heat to low and simmer for 25-35 minutes, partially covered, until lentils are tender. Add spinach and continue cooking for 5 minutes or until spinach is wilted.

Grapes or other fruit for dessert

> **Tip:** Note the sodium content of the packaged foods you purchase—you'll be surprised to see how much sodium is in the products you use every day. Choose foods that are labeled "no salt added" or "low sodium." If you use canned beans, select no-salt-added varieties.

> **Tip:** To water sauté, heat a tablespoon or two of water in a pan, wok or skillet. When hot, add the vegetables and cook, covering occasionally and adding additional liquid as needed until the vegetables are tender. Don't add too much water or the vegetables will be boiled, not sautéed.

DINNER

VERY VEGGIE BURRITOS
4 SERVINGS

1 red or green bell pepper, seeded and cored
1 medium onion, cut into wedges

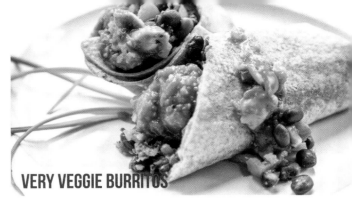
VERY VEGGIE BURRITOS

1 cup chopped mushrooms
3 cloves garlic
1 cup packed chopped kale
2 cups cooked or no-salt-added canned red or black beans, drained
1 ½ cups diced tomatoes
1 cup shredded carrots
1 ½ cups low sodium salsa, divided
2-3 teaspoons chili powder
1 teaspoon cumin
¼ teaspoon red pepper flakes, or to taste
8 (100 percent whole grain) tortillas or 1 head romaine or other leafy lettuce
½ avocado, peeled and pitted

Chop and combine bell pepper, onion, mushrooms, garlic and kale in a food processor. Remove from food processor and sauté mixture in a small amount of water until veggies are very tender.

Add beans, tomatoes, carrots, ½ cup of the salsa and spices. Stir and simmer until most of the tomato liquid evaporates. Remove from heat.

Blend or mash together the remaining cup of salsa with the avocado. Spoon beans and veggies onto lettuce leaves or tortillas, top with salsa/avocado mixture and roll tightly.

Your choice of a cooked green or high-nutrient, non-green vegetable
The high-nutrient, non-green vegetables are: tomatoes, onions, mushrooms, cauliflower, eggplant and red peppers.

Melon or other fruit for dessert

DAY 4

You need to rethink portion sizes and learn to consume larger amounts of the right foods. The more raw and cooked vegetables you eat, the better.

BREAKFAST

BLUEBERRY ALMOND SALAD
1 SERVING

1 banana
½ cup unsweetened soy, hemp or almond milk
1 tablespoon raw almond butter
1 teaspoon ground flax seeds
1 cup fresh or thawed frozen blueberries (or other berries)
2 cups shredded romaine lettuce
2 tablespoons chopped almonds

Blend banana, non-dairy milk, almond butter and flax seeds in a high-powered blender until smooth. Place berries on a bed of shredded lettuce and top with the almond sauce and chopped almonds.

> **Tip:** If you are still hungry, see the list of Foods to Eat Liberally on page 19.

LUNCH

GREEN SALAD WITH TOMATO MUSTARD DRESSING
(or leftover Strawberry Almond Balsamic from Day 2)

Include mixed greens, tomatoes, red onions and raw sunflower or pumpkin seeds in your salad.

To make Tomato Mustard Dressing, whisk together ⅓ cup no-salt-added tomato sauce, 2 tablespoons raw cashew butter, 2 teaspoons balsamic vinegar, 2 teaspoons mustard and 1 teaspoon water.

BROCCOLI QUICHE WITH AQUAFABA
4 SERVINGS

1 large onion, sliced
1 cup chopped mushrooms
5 cups small broccoli florets
14 ounces firm tofu, drained
½ cup chickpea aquafaba (see note)
¼ cup unsweetened soy, hemp or almond milk
¼ cup nutritional yeast
2 tablespoons raw cashew butter
2 tablespoons arrowroot powder
1 teaspoon Bragg Liquid Aminos or reduced-sodium soy sauce
1 teaspoon paprika
1 teaspoon Dijon mustard
½ teaspoon garlic powder
½ teaspoon turmeric
¼ teaspoon ground black pepper

Preheat oven to 375 degrees F.

Heat 2-3 tablespoons of water in a large pan and add onion and mushrooms. Water sauté until onions are tender, adding small amounts of additional water as needed to prevent sticking. Add broccoli and a few more tablespoons of water, cover and cook until broccoli is almost tender, about five minutes.

Combine remaining ingredients in a high-powered blender and blend for at least one minute to whip up the aquafaba.

Place broccoli mixture in an eight-inch cake pan that has been wiped with olive oil. Pour blended mixture on top and stir to combine. Bake for 35-40 minutes or until top is golden brown. Allow to cool for 10 minutes before cutting.

Note: Aquafaba is the cooking liquid from beans and other legumes like chickpeas. It is the typically discarded liquid found in retail cans and boxes of beans, or the liquid left over from cooking your own dried beans. Save the drained chickpeas! You will use them for your salad tomorrow.

Apple or other fresh or frozen fruit for dessert

> **Tip:** If you are invited to a get-together where there may be no healthy food choices, bring your own dish plus extra to share with others. Try to eat something healthful before you go, so you don't arrive hungry and tempted to overindulge.

DINNER

CREAMY WHITE BEAN AND KALE SOUP
4 SERVINGS

8 large garlic cloves, minced
1 medium onion, chopped
2 cups sliced mushrooms
8 cups chopped kale
8 cups no-salt-added vegetable broth, divided
4 ½ cups cooked or 3 (15 ounce) cans no-salt-added white beans, drained, divided
4 plum tomatoes, chopped
1 teaspoon dried oregano
½ teaspoon dried basil
½ teaspoon dried thyme
½ cup chopped fresh parsley
black pepper, to taste

In a large pot, heat 2-3 tablespoons of vegetable broth and sauté garlic, onion and mushrooms until soft. Add kale, 6 cups of the vegetable broth, 2 cups of the beans, tomatoes, herbs and pepper. Simmer for 5 minutes.

In a blender or food processor, blend the remaining broth and beans until smooth. Stir into the soup. Simmer for 30 minutes or until kale is very tender.

Refrigerate leftover soup or freeze in individual containers to enjoy as an alternative lunch or dinner.

TOMATO SALAD

Mix together chopped tomatoes, chopped cucumbers, chopped red onion and basil leaves. Sprinkle with balsamic vinegar and season with oregano and black pepper.

Pineapple chunks and chopped orange segments sprinkled with unsweetened shredded coconut for dessert

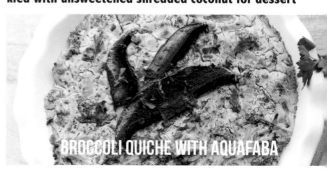

BROCCOLI QUICHE WITH AQUAFABA

DAY 5

Nuts and seeds have been linked to protection from cardiovascular disease in hundreds of studies. Eating five or more servings of nuts per week is estimated to reduce the risk of heart disease by 35 percent.

BREAKFAST

GOOD FOR YOU GRANOLA BARS
9 SERVINGS

3 ripe bananas
½ Granny Smith apple, chopped into small pieces
1 cup raisins
1 cup chopped walnuts
½ cup raw sunflower seeds
¼ cup unhulled sesame seeds
1 teaspoon cinnamon or pumpkin pie spice
2 cups old-fashioned oats

Preheat oven to 300 degrees F. Mash bananas to a soft consistency. Add remaining ingredients. Add a small amount of non-dairy milk, if needed, to help mixing.

Lightly oil a 9x9 inch baking dish. Pour mixture into dish and press to a firm consistency. Bake mixture for 40 minutes. Remove from oven, let cool, then cut into bars.

Wrap bars individually and store in the refrigerator or freezer. They can be used as an alternative breakfast when you are short on time. Limit to 1 per day.

VANILLA HEMP-ALMOND MILK
2 SERVINGS

2 ½ cups water
¼ cup hemp seeds
¼ cup raw almonds
1 Medjool or 2 regular dates, pitted
½ teaspoon alcohol-free vanilla extract or ground vanilla bean powder

Blend all ingredients in a high-powered blender until smooth.

LUNCH

ROASTED BEETS WITH LEAFY GREENS, RED ONIONS AND WALNUTS
2 SERVINGS

2 medium red or golden beets
¼ cup apple cider vinegar
2 tablespoons raisins, finely chopped (or use dried currants)
1 tablespoon toasted caraway seeds, chopped
1 teaspoon garlic, finely chopped
10 cups Boston or green leaf lettuce
⅓ medium red onion, thinly sliced
¼ cup chopped walnuts

Roast beets at 350 degrees F for 50-60 minutes, or until tender when pierced. Let cool and peel off the skins. Slice thinly.

Whisk together the red wine vinegar, chopped raisins, toasted caraway seeds and chopped garlic. Add sliced beets and marinate for 1 hour.

In a large salad bowl, toss beet and vinegar mixture with remaining ingredients.

Lightly steamed green beans or other cooked green vegetable (or leftover Creamy White Bean and Kale Soup)

Grapes or other fruit for dessert

DINNER

THAI BRAISED KALE WITH TOFU (OR CHICKEN OR SHRIMP)
4 SERVINGS

14 ounces firm tofu, drained well, cut into 1-inch cubes (see note)
1 cup finely chopped onion
1 tablespoon grated fresh ginger
1 small jalapeño pepper, seeded and minced
2 cups sliced mushrooms
1 teaspoon chili powder
2 cups no-salt-added vegetable broth
½ cup no-salt-added, natural peanut butter
2 tablespoons tomato paste
2 tablespoons Dr. Fuhrman's MatoZest (or other no-salt seasoning blend, adjusted to taste)
1 bunch kale, tough stems and center ribs removed and leaves chopped
1 tablespoon fresh lime juice
4 scallions, thinly sliced

Preheat oven to 350 degrees F. Place tofu cubes on a lightly-oiled baking dish and bake for 30 minutes, turning after 15 minutes.

Heat a large sauté pan and add onion, ginger, jalapeño and mushrooms. Cook until onion has softened, adding 1-2 teaspoons of water as needed to prevent sticking. Add chili powder and cook one more minute.

Whisk in vegetable broth, peanut butter, tomato paste, MatoZest and bring to a boil. Gradually add kale a few handfuls at a time, stirring to let it wilt down. Add baked tofu, cover, reduce heat, and simmer for 10 minutes or until kale is tender. Stir in lime juice and top with sliced scallions.

Note: If you like, make the recipe without baked tofu and top with 2 ounces of cooked shrimp or shredded chicken per serving.

Cooked wild rice (1 cup per serving)
Blueberries or other fresh or frozen berries

Tip: If you choose to include animal products in your diet, use them only in small amounts to add flavor. They should not exceed 6 ounces per week or 2 ounces per serving. Avoid eating red meat, processed meats and full-fat dairy.

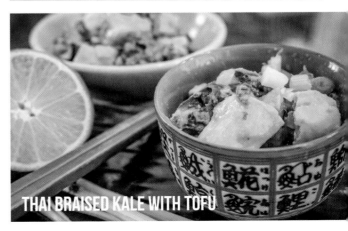

THAI BRAISED KALE WITH TOFU

DAYS 6-10
SHOPPING LIST

This shopping list assumes that all recipes in the meal plan will be made. Menus frequently include fruit for dessert and will mention a specific fruit as an example. That fruit is used for the shopping list.

Check your refrigerator, freezer and pantry before shopping. You may have items leftover from Days 1-5 that you can use. Make sure you also have all the items listed in the Stock Your Pantry list.

FRESH PRODUCE

VEGETABLES

- [ ] 2 heads romaine lettuce
- [ ] Mixed baby greens (need 2 cups)
- [ ] 7 ounces arugula (need 10 cups)
- [ ] 2 bunches kale
- [ ] 15 ounces spinach
- [ ] 1 small green cabbage
- [ ] 1 small Napa cabbage
- [ ] 1 endive
- [ ] Broccoli (about 2 cups of florets)
- [ ] 1 head cauliflower
- [ ] 1 bunch asparagus
- [ ] Your choice of a green leafy vegetable such as kale, collards or Swiss chard to equal 2 cups cooked (could also buy frozen)
- [ ] Your choice of a green vegetable such as broccoli, asparagus or green beans to equal 2 cups cooked (could also buy frozen)
- [ ] 3 red bell peppers
- [ ] 1 jalapeno pepper
- [ ] Snow peas (need 1 cup)
- [ ] 1 cucumber
- [ ] Carrots (need 1)
- [ ] 4 tomatoes
- [ ] Pint of cherry or grape tomatoes
- [ ] 25 ounces white or cremini mushrooms
- [ ] Shiitake mushrooms (need 3 cups)
- [ ] 2 avocados
- [ ] 3 sweet potatoes
- [ ] 3 yellow onions
- [ ] 2 red onions
- [ ] Scallions (need 10)
- [ ] Radishes
- [ ] 2 inch-piece of ginger (any left from Days 1-5?)
- [ ] 1 bulb garlic
- [ ] Cilantro
- [ ] Basil

FRUIT

- [ ] 2 cups blueberries (could be frozen)
- [ ] 2 cups raspberries (could be frozen)
- [ ] 3 oranges
- [ ] Small bunch of grapes (need 1 cup)
- [ ] 2 apples
- [ ] 1 pear
- [ ] 1 mango
- [ ] Pineapple (need about 2 cups)
- [ ] 4 bananas
- [ ] 2 lemons
- [ ] 1 lime

REFRIGERATED

- [ ] 6 ¼ cups unsweetened unflavored soy, hemp or almond milk
- [ ] 1 (14 ounce) package firm tofu
- [ ] 1 (14 ounce) package extra-firm tofu
- [ ] Hummus (If you choose to make your own, add the ingredients in the Day 9 Lunch hummus recipe to your shopping list.)
- [ ] 1 cup pomegranate juice

FROZEN

This list does not include vegetables and fruit listed under fresh produce that have a frozen option.

- [ ] Strawberries (need 2 cups) any left from Days 1-5?
- [ ] Blueberries (need 1 cup)
- [ ] Cherries (need 2 cups), could also buy fresh
- [ ] Peaches (need 2 cups)
- [ ] Edamame in the pod

SHELF STABLE

BEANS

It is assumed that canned beans will be used. Select no-salt-added varieties. If you opt to start with dry beans, 1 cup of dry beans will yield about 3 cups of cooked beans.

- [ ] 1 (15 ounce) can cannellini or other white beans
- [ ] 1 (15 ounce) can black beans
- [ ] 2 (15 ounce) cans chickpeas

OTHER

Choose tomato products packaged in BPA-free materials.

- [ ] 4 ½ cups no-salt-added vegetable broth
- [ ] Low-sodium salsa (need about ½ cup) If you choose to make your own, add the ingredients in the Day 6 Lunch salsa recipe to your shopping list.
- [ ] No-salt-added or low-sodium pasta sauce (need 1 cup)
- [ ] No-salt-added tomato sauce (need 1/3 cup)
- [ ] No-salt-added tomato paste (need 2 tablespoons)
- [ ] Bean pasta (such as Tolerant brand)
- [ ] Chipotle chili powder
- [ ] Low-sodium miso paste
- [ ] White balsamic vinegar

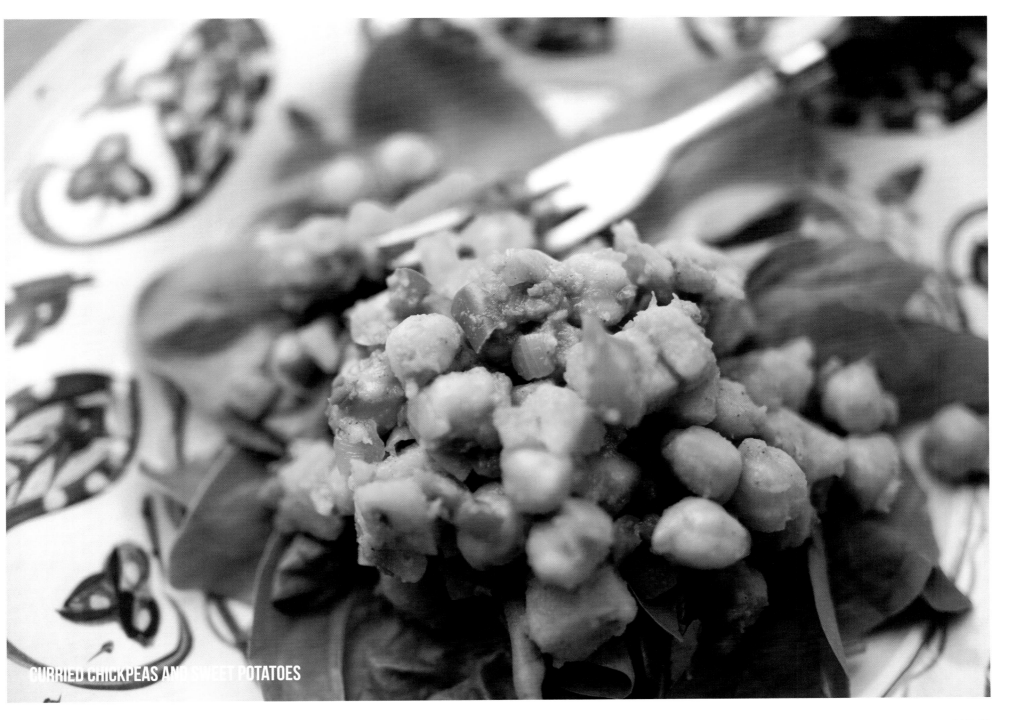

CURRIED CHICKPEAS AND SWEET POTATOES

DAY 6

Salt is simply sodium chloride—and no matter what marketers call it, or what it costs, or what trendy claims are made about it, the truth is, it's bad for you. The human body was designed to get its optimal level of sodium from a natural diet, but most Americans consume about six times what they need.

BREAKFAST

BLUEBERRY NUT STEEL-CUT OATS
1 SERVING

1 cup water
¼ cup steel-cut oats
½ cup diced apple
1 tablespoon ground flax seeds
½ cup fresh or frozen blueberries
2 tablespoons chopped walnuts or pecans

In a saucepan, bring water to a boil and stir in all ingredients, except blueberries and nuts. Reduce heat, cover, and simmer for 15 minutes or until oats are tender and water is absorbed, stirring occasionally.

Stir in blueberries, heat for another minute or two. Remove from heat and stir in nuts.

> **Tip:** Steel-cut oats are less processed than other forms of oats. They are simply oat kernels that have been chopped into pieces.

LUNCH

CHIPOTLE, AVOCADO, AND WHITE BEAN WRAPS
2 SERVINGS

½ cup raw pumpkin seeds
¼ cup apple cider vinegar
½ cup unsweetened soy, hemp or almond milk

¼ cup raisins
2 cups shredded red cabbage
1 medium carrot, peeled and shredded
2 tablespoons chopped fresh cilantro
1 cup cooked or no-salt-added canned white beans, drained
½ ripe avocado, peeled
2 tablespoons minced red onion
¼ teaspoon chipotle chili powder or more to taste
2 (100 percent whole grain) flour tortillas (see note)

In a high-powered blender, blend pumpkin seeds to a fine powder. Add vinegar, non-dairy milk and raisins and process until smooth. Combine cabbage, carrot and cilantro and toss with desired amount of dressing.

Mash beans and avocado together with a fork. Stir in red onion and chipotle chili powder.

To assemble the wraps, spread about 1/2 cup bean/avocado mixture onto each wrap, and top with cabbage mixture. Roll up.

Note: For a gluten-free option, toss dressing with chopped romaine in addition to the cabbage, carrot and cilantro and top with bean and avocado mixture.

Save leftover dressing, you can use it as a sauce for your cooked vegetable at dinner. Save leftover beans, you can use them for your lunch salad on Day 8.

ENDIVE LEAVES WITH LOW-SODIUM SALSA

To make your own salsa, mix together 2 chopped tomatoes, 1 small chopped red onion, 1 clove minced garlic, ½ chopped jalapeño, 3 tablespoons cilantro and 3 tablespoons lime juice.

Orange or other fresh or frozen fruit for dessert

DINNER

CURRIED CHICKPEAS AND SWEET POTATOES
2 SERVINGS

2 sweet potatoes, peeled and diced
⅓ cup no-salt-added vegetable broth
1 red bell pepper, diced
1 small onion, diced
1 tablespoon minced fresh ginger
1 clove garlic, minced
1 teaspoon no-salt seasoning, adjusted to taste
1 tablespoon curry powder
1 ½ cups cooked or 1 (15 ounce) can no-salt-added chickpeas, drained
1 teaspoon apple cider vinegar

Steam sweet potatoes in a large saucepan filled with an inch of water and fitted with a steamer basket for 10 minutes or until cooked through. Set aside and keep warm.

In another large pot, heat ⅓ cup vegetable broth and stir in pepper, onion, ginger, garlic, no-salt seasoning and curry powder. Stir, cover, and cook for 3-5 minutes or until vegetables are tender. Add chickpeas and simmer uncovered for 5 minutes. Add vinegar and sweet potatoes and heat for a few more minutes, stirring gently. Add additional water or vegetable broth, if needed, to adjust consistency.

Your choice of a steamed or water-sautéed green, leafy vegetable such as kale, collards or Swiss chard (can be fresh or frozen).

> **Tip:** Water sauté vegetables with fresh chopped garlic or onion. Season with lemon, balsamic vinegar and/or your choice of herbs, spices or a no-salt seasoning blend.

STRAWBERRY BANANA ICE CREAM
4 SERVINGS

3 ripe bananas, frozen

⅓ cup unsweetened soy, hemp or almond milk

2 cups frozen strawberries (see note)

2 tablespoons chopped walnuts

1 tablespoon ground flax seed

½ teaspoon alcohol-free vanilla extract or pure
  vanilla bean powder

Blend all ingredients in a high-powered blender until smooth
and creamy. Add additional non-dairy milk, if needed, to
adjust consistency.

Note: For Blueberry Banana Ice Cream, substitute
frozen blueberries.

*Portion leftover ice cream into individual servings and freeze.
Enjoy with another meal.*

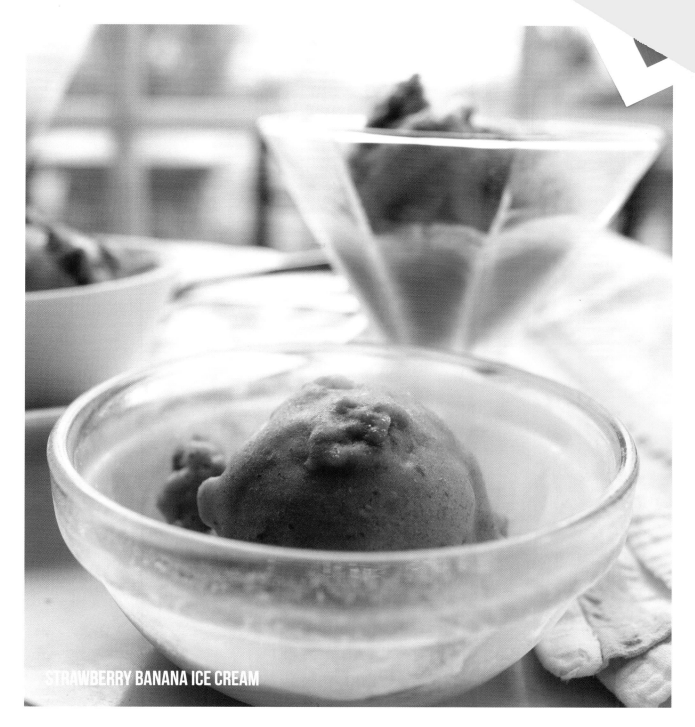

STRAWBERRY BANANA ICE CREAM

DAY 7

To achieve optimal health, there is no escaping the fact that you must significantly reduce or eliminate the consumption of animal products.

BREAKFAST

QUINOA BREAKFAST PUDDING
4 SERVINGS

¾ cup quinoa, rinsed
3 cups water
8 regular or 4 Medjool dates, pitted
2 cups unsweetened soy, hemp or almond milk
1 teaspoon alcohol-free vanilla extract
¼ cup slivered almonds or coarsely ground walnuts
½ cup raisins or currants
1 cup finely chopped spinach
1 cup finely chopped kale leaves
⅛ teaspoon cinnamon

Preheat oven to 350 degrees F. In a large saucepan, bring quinoa and 3 cups water to a boil. Reduce heat and simmer, uncovered, until grains are translucent and the mixture is the consistency of a thick porridge, about 20 minutes.

In a high-powered blender, blend dates, non-dairy milk and vanilla. Add this mixture to the cooked quinoa. Stir in the nuts, currants, spinach and kale. Pour mixture into a lightly-oiled 9x9 inch baking dish and sprinkle with cinnamon. Bake for 30 minutes. Serve warm or cold.

Fresh or frozen cherries or other fruit

LUNCH

KALE AND FRUIT SALAD
2 SERVINGS
For the Dressing:

¼ cup raw almonds
2 oranges, juiced
2 teaspoons balsamic vinegar
6 large chunks fresh pineapple
For the Salad:
6 cups kale, finely chopped
1 apple, chopped
1 cup grapes, whole or sliced
1 cup fresh mango chunks

Combine the dressing ingredients in a high-powered blender. Toss desired amount of dressing with the salad ingredients. Leftover dressing can be refrigerated for another use.

Edamame sprinkled with nutritional yeast and salt-free seasoning

DINNER

Mixed Green Salad with Creamy Lemon Dressing
Include romaine, spinach, tomato and scallions in your salad.

CREAMY LEMON SALAD DRESSING
6 SERVINGS

1 cup unsweetened soy, hemp or almond milk
½ cup raw cashews
½ cup hemp seeds
1 large lemon, juiced
2 teaspoons mustard
2 cloves garlic, minced
½ cup Dr. Fuhrman's Riesling Reserve Vinegar or other flavored vinegar

Blend ingredients in a high-powered blender until very smooth.

Leftover dressing can be used as a veggie dip for tomorrow's dinner.

PESTO PIZZA WITH BROCCOLI, MUSHROOMS AND ONIONS
4 SERVINGS

For the Pesto:
2 cloves garlic
½ cup walnuts
¼ cup balsamic vinegar

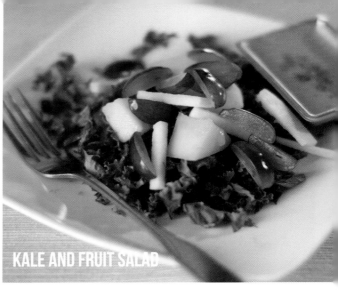

KALE AND FRUIT SALAD

1-2 teaspoons lemon juice or to taste
½ cup water
½ tablespoon Dr. Fuhrman's MatoZest (or other no-salt Italian seasoning, adjusted to taste)
½ tablespoon nutritional yeast
2 cups arugula
2 cups spinach

To Assemble the Pizza:
1 large red onion, sliced
10 ounces mushrooms, sliced
2 cups small broccoli florets
4 (100% whole grain) flour tortillas or pitas
1 medium tomato, chopped

To make the pesto, add the garlic, walnuts, vinegar, lemon juice, water, MatoZest and nutritional yeast to a food processor or blender and blend at high speed. Turn to low speed and add the arugula and spinach and blend to a chunky consistency. Set aside.

Preheat oven to 350 degrees F. Heat 2-3 tablespoons water in a large pan and sauté red onion for 1-2 minutes, add mushrooms and broccoli and continue to cook until onions and broccoli are tender and liquid from mushrooms has cooked off.

Bake tortillas or pitas directly on oven rack for 5-7 minutes or until just crisp. Spread a thin layer of pesto sauce on each tortilla or pita bread and top with the sautéed vegetable mixture and tomato. Bake for an additional 3-5 minutes or until toppings are warm, checking occasionally to avoid browning of vegetables.

If you are following a gluten-free diet, substitute a dinner item from another night.

DAY 8

Green leafy vegetables are as close to a miracle food as we can get. These vegetables are powerfully associated with a lower risk of death from cardiovascular disease and all other causes.

BREAKFAST
MADISON TOFU SCRAMBLE
2 SERVINGS

3 whole scallions, diced
½ cup finely chopped red bell pepper
1 medium tomato, chopped
2 cloves garlic, minced or pressed
1 ½ cups mushrooms, small slices or diced
14 ounces firm tofu, drained and crumbled
½ teaspoon Mrs. Dash or other no-salt seasoning blend
1 tablespoon nutritional yeast
1 teaspoon cumin
½ teaspoon ground turmeric
5 ounces spinach, coarsely chopped
1 teaspoon Bragg Liquid Aminos or low-sodium soy sauce

In a large skillet, over medium/high heat, sauté scallions, red pepper, tomato and garlic in ¼ cup water for 5 minutes. Add remaining ingredients and cook for another 5 to 8 minutes.

Sliced avocado (about ¼ avocado per serving)

LUNCH

Big Green Salad with Walnut Vinaigrette Dressing

Include romaine lettuce, shredded cabbage, tomatoes, red onions, ½ cup any variety beans, and pumpkin seeds in your salad.

> **Tip:** Remember to add some cruciferous vegetables into your raw green salads: shredded red or green cabbage, baby kale, arugula, watercress, Chinese cabbage or bok choy.

WALNUT VINAIGRETTE DRESSING
4 SERVINGS

¼ cup balsamic vinegar
½ cup water
¼ cup walnuts
¼ cup raisins
1 teaspoon Dijon mustard
1 clove garlic
¼ teaspoon dried thyme

Combine all ingredients in a high-powered blender.

TOFU BITES
2 SERVINGS

Cut extra-firm tofu (14-ounce box) into thin slices and place on a wire rack. Mix 1 cup low-sodium pasta sauce, 2 tablespoons tomato paste, 1 teaspoon garlic powder and 1 teaspoon onion powder and spread over the tofu. Bake in a 225 degree F oven for 60 minutes or until tofu is yellowed on the outside.

Raspberries or other berries topped with ground flax seeds for dessert

DINNER
CAULIFLOWER SOUP WITH COCONUT, GINGER AND TURMERIC
4 SERVINGS

½ cup unsweetened shredded coconut
1 teaspoon chopped fresh ginger
1 cup water
1 medium onion, chopped
4 cloves garlic, chopped
3 cups sliced shiitake mushrooms
1 head cauliflower, cut into pieces
4 ½ cups no-salt-added vegetable broth
½ teaspoon ground turmeric
½ teaspoon ground coriander
¾ cup raw cashews
1 bunch kale, tough stems removed, chopped

Blend coconut, ginger and water in a high-powered blender until smooth and creamy.

In a soup pot, heat 2-3 tablespoons water and water sauté onion and garlic for two minutes, then add mushrooms, onions and mushrooms are tender. Add blended coconut, cauliflower, vegetable broth, turmeric and coriander. boil, reduce heat, cover and simmer for 15 minutes or cauliflower is tender.

Blend two-thirds of the soup liquid and vegetables with the cashews in a high-powered blender until smooth and creamy. Return to the pot.

Steam the kale until wilted and just tender, about 6-8 minutes. Divide some of the steamed kale in a soup bowl and pour the soup on top

Steamed Asparagus or other fresh or frozen green vegetable

CHICKPEA POPCORN
3 SERVINGS

To make Chickpea Popcorn, preheat oven to 325 degrees F. Mix 1 ½ cups cooked chickpeas with 1 teaspoon cumin, 1 teaspoon garlic powder, 1 teaspoon oregano, a pinch of cayenne pepper and 1 teaspoon of olive oil. Spread on a baking sheet and bake for 45 minutes or until crispy, stirring occasionally.

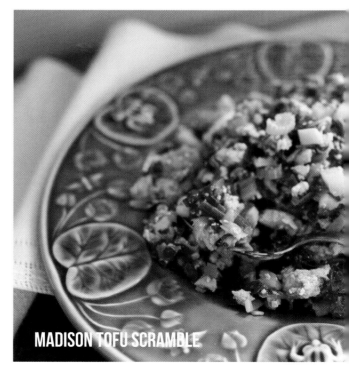

MADISON TOFU SCRAMBLE

DAY 9

Avoid empty-calorie foods such as sugar, sweeteners, white flour, processed foods and fast foods. They fuel addictive food behaviors and have no nutritional value.

BREAKFAST

PURPLE POWER SMOOTHIE
1 SERVING

1 cup pomegranate juice
2 cups kale, tough stems removed, coarsely chopped
¼ medium cucumber
1 cup frozen blueberries or mixed berries
2 regular or 1 Medjool date, pitted
1 tablespoon ground flax seeds

Blend ingredients in high-powered blender until smooth and creamy.

BANANA NUT LETTUCE WRAPS
1 SERVING

2 tablespoons raw cashew or almond butter
6 romaine lettuce leaves
1 banana, thinly sliced

Spread some nut butter on each lettuce leaf. Lay a few banana slices on top and roll up.

LUNCH

MEDITERRANEAN FARRO SALAD
(or leftover Cauliflower Soup from Day 8 dinner)
4 SERVINGS

1 cup farro
2 ½ cups water
4 cups arugula

¾ cup halved cherry or grape tomatoes
¼ cup thinly sliced radishes
⅓ cup fresh basil, torn
¼ cup pine nuts or chopped walnuts

For the Dressing:
⅓ cup no-salt-added tomato sauce
2 tablespoons raw cashew butter
2 teaspoons balsamic vinegar
1 teaspoon mustard
1 tablespoon water

In a medium saucepan, bring farro and water to a boil, reduce heat, cover and simmer until the farro is tender, about 20 minutes. Drain well, transfer to a large bowl and let cool. Add arugula, tomatoes, radishes, basil and nuts.

Whisk together tomato sauce, cashew butter, balsamic vinegar, mustard and water until smooth. Add to farro mixture and toss to combine.

RAW VEGETABLES WITH HUMMUS

To make oil-free, no-salt-added hummus, blend 1 ½ cups cooked chickpeas, 2 tablespoons lemon juice, 2 tablespoons unhulled sesame seeds, 1 garlic clove and ½ teaspoon cumin in a food processor or high-powered blender. Add 1-2 tablespoons water if needed to adjust consistency

Pear or other fruit for dessert

> **Tip:** Grain products are not as nutrient dense as vegetables and fruit so they should make up a smaller portion of your diet. Choose intact whole grains that have not been ground up such as steel-cut oats, buckwheat, quinoa, farro, freekeh or wild rice.

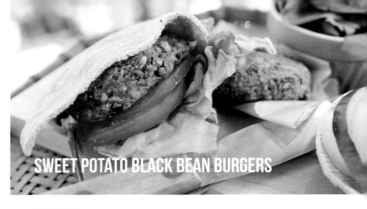

SWEET POTATO BLACK BEAN BURGERS

DINNER

SWEET POTATO BLACK BEAN BURGERS
6 SERVINGS

½ cup raw almonds
1 ½ cups cooked or 1 (15 ounce) can no-salt-added black beans, drained
¾ cup baked sweet potato, mashed
½ cup diced red onion
½ jalapeño pepper, deseeded and diced
3 tablespoons chopped cilantro
1 teaspoon garlic powder
½ teaspoon black pepper
2 teaspoons apple cider vinegar
1 tablespoon fresh lime juice
3 tablespoons nutritional yeast
old-fashioned oats or 100 percent whole grain bread crumbs, if needed, to adjust consistency

Place almonds in a food processor and grind to a fine powder. Add remaining ingredients except for oats and pulse to combine.

Form mixture into 6 burgers. If mixture is too wet, a small amount of oats or whole grain bread crumbs may be added. Place on a lightly-oiled or parchment-lined baking sheet. Bake at 350 degrees for 30 minutes or until lightly browned.

Serve with sliced tomato, avocado and onion on a 100 percent whole grain pita (cut open to make 2 flat pieces) or on a bed of greens. (If using a pita, have one burger; have two if serving on greens.)

Wrap leftover burgers individually and freeze. They work well as a quick on-the-run lunch or dinner.

Thawed, frozen peaches with fresh or frozen raspberries or other fruit for dessert

DAY 10

Across a variety of different regions and ethnicities, beans have been found to be the most consistent and reliable predictor of longevity. Eating more beans as a replacement for other foods aids in all metabolic parameters that enhance cardiovascular health.

BREAKFAST

SCRAMBLED OATS
2 SERVINGS

1 cup steel-cut oats (see note)
2 cups water (or no-salt-added or low-sodium vegetable broth)
1 tablespoon nutritional yeast
1 teaspoon reduced-sodium miso paste
½ teaspoon ground turmeric
2 cups fresh spinach or other leafy greens
1 cup lightly sautéed sliced mushrooms
grated red or yellow onion for garnish

Combine oats, water, nutritional yeast, miso and turmeric in a saucepan and cook, stirring frequently, for about 20 minutes or until oats are tender. Stir in spinach and mushrooms and cook until spinach is wilted. Garnish with grated onion.

Note: You may also use old-fashioned oats in this recipe. Reduce cooking time to 5 minutes.

Halved cherry or grape tomatoes

LUNCH

NAPA CABBAGE SALAD WITH SESAME PEANUT DRESSING
2 SERVINGS

For the Dressing:
¼ cup no-salt-added natural peanut butter

2 tablespoons unhulled sesame seeds
¼ cup unsweetened soy, hemp or almond milk
¼ cup water
¼ cup rice vinegar
3 regular or 1 ½ Medjool dates, pitted
1 clove garlic, chopped
1 tablespoon chopped fresh ginger
1 teaspoon Bragg Liquid Aminos or low-sodium soy sauce

For the Salad:
4 cups shredded Napa cabbage
4 cups shredded romaine lettuce
1 small red bell pepper, thinly sliced
1 cup thinly-sliced snow peas
4 scallions, sliced

Blend dressing ingredients in a high-powered blender until smooth.

Combine salad ingredients in a large bowl and toss with desired amount of dressing.

Sweet Potato Black Bean Burger (leftover from Day 9 dinner, serve without the pita) or add ½-1 cup of beans to the Napa Cabbage Salad

Fresh or frozen blueberries or other berries for dessert

DINNER

Bean pasta with Arugula Pesto

ARUGULA PESTO
4 SERVINGS

2 cloves garlic
½ cup walnuts
¼ cup white balsamic vinegar
½ cup water
½ tablespoon Dr. Fuhrman's VegiZest (or other no-salt seasoning blend, adjusted to taste)
½ tablespoon nutritional yeast
2 cups arugula
2 cups spinach

Add the garlic, walnuts, vinegar, water, VegiZest and nutritional yeast to a high-powered blender and blend at high speed. Turn the blender to low speed and add the arugula and spinach and blend to a chunky consistency.

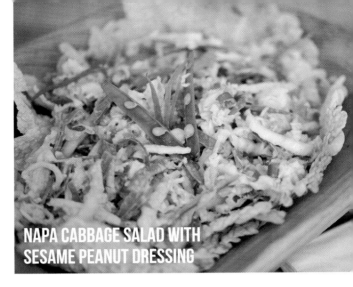

NAPA CABBAGE SALAD WITH SESAME PEANUT DRESSING

Note: Any combination of greens and nuts may be used.

Your choice of a steamed or water-sautéed green vegetable (can be fresh or frozen)

Tip: Bean Pasta is available in different shapes and is made from different kinds of beans. If you can't find bean pasta, use thinly sliced or spiralized zucchini.

CHOCOLATE CHIA PUDDING
4 SERVINGS

2 cups unsweetened soy, hemp or almond milk
8 regular or 4 Medjool dates, pitted
3 tablespoons natural cocoa powder
½ teaspoon alcohol-free vanilla extract or pure vanilla bean powder
½ cup chia seeds
raspberries or other berries

Blend non-dairy milk, dates, cocoa powder, vanilla and 2 tablespoons of the chia seeds in a high-powered blender. Stir in remaining chia seeds. Refrigerate for 15 minutes and stir again to distribute seeds evenly.

Top with berries.

Refrigerate leftover pudding and enjoy it as a dessert or breakfast over the next few days.

DAYS 11-15
SHOPPING LIST

This shopping list assumes that all recipes in the meal plan will be made. Menus frequently include fruit for dessert and will mention a specific fruit as an example. That fruit is used for the shopping list.

Check your refrigerator, freezer and pantry before shopping. You may have items leftover from Days 1-10 that you can use. Make sure you also have all the items listed in the Stock Your Pantry list.

FRESH PRODUCE
VEGETABLES
- [ ] 3 heads romaine lettuce
- [ ] 12 ounces mixed baby greens (about 12 cups)
- [ ] 2 bunches kale
- [ ] 14 ounces spinach (12 ounces could be frozen)
- [ ] 1 bunch Swiss chard
- [ ] Red cabbage (need about 1 cup)
- [ ] Green cabbage (need 1 ½ cups)
- [ ] 1 head cauliflower
- [ ] Broccoli (about 2 cups florets)
- [ ] Your choice of green vegetable equal to 2 cups cooked (could also buy frozen)
- [ ] Raw vegetables of choice to eat with dip
- [ ] 7 red bell peppers
- [ ] 2 jalapeno peppers
- [ ] 2 red chili peppers
- [ ] 5 cucumbers
- [ ] Carrots (need 2)
- [ ] Celery (4 stalks)

- [ ] 7 tomatoes
- [ ] White or cremini mushrooms (need 1 cup sliced)
- [ ] 2 large Portobello mushrooms
- [ ] 7 ounces shiitake mushrooms (if not having salmon on Day 15)
- [ ] 2 avocados
- [ ] 9 ears of corn (could also use 5 cups frozen corn kernels)
- [ ] 2 eggplants
- [ ] 1 spaghetti squash
- [ ] 1 yellow squash
- [ ] 1 zucchini
- [ ] 1 butternut squash (need 4 cups chopped)
- [ ] 6 yellow onions
- [ ] 1 white sweet onion
- [ ] 1 red onion
- [ ] Radishes (need 2)
- [ ] Scallions (need 2)
- [ ] 1 head garlic
- [ ] Cilantro
- [ ] Parsley
- [ ] Dill (could also use dry)

FRUIT
- [ ] Raspberries and/or blackberries (need about 4 cups)
- [ ] 2 ½ cups blueberries (could be frozen)
- [ ] 1 cup organic strawberries (could use frozen which do not need to be organic)
- [ ] 1 orange
- [ ] 2 clementines
- [ ] Small bunch of grapes
- [ ] 1 melon, any variety
- [ ] 3 apples
- [ ] 1 pear
- [ ] Pineapple (need about 2 cups)
- [ ] 2 bananas
- [ ] 3 limes

REFRIGERATED
- [ ] 3 cups unsweetened, unflavored soy, hemp or almond milk
- [ ] ⅓ cup pomegranate juice (any left from Days 6-10?)
- [ ] Carrot juice (need ⅓ cup)

- [ ] Low-sodium hummus (If you choose to make your own, add the ingredients in the Day 12 Lunch hummus recipe to your shopping list.)
- [ ] 4 ounces extra-firm tofu
- [ ] 4 ounces wild-caught salmon, optional

FROZEN
This list does not include vegetables and fruit listed under fresh produce that have a frozen option.
- [ ] Cherries (need 3 cups)
- [ ] Shelled edamame (need 1 cup)

SHELF STABLE
BEANS
It is assumed that canned beans will be used. Select no-salt-added varieties. If you opt to start with dry beans, 1 cup of dry beans will yield about 3 cups of cooked beans
- [ ] 3 (15 ounce) cans black beans
- [ ] 2 (15 ounce) cans chickpeas
- [ ] 1 (15 ounce) can pinto beans
- [ ] 1 (15 ounce) can black beans

OTHER
Choose tomato products packaged in BPA-free materials.
- [ ] 2 (32 ounce) cartons no-salt-added vegetable broth
- [ ] ½ cup low-sodium salsa (Could also make your own or just use chopped, fresh tomatoes. If you choose to make your own salsa, add the ingredients in the Day 11 Breakfast salsa recipe to your shopping list.)
- [ ] No-salt-added diced tomatoes (need 3 cups)
- [ ] No-salt-added or low-sodium pasta sauce (need 2 ½ cups)
- [ ] 1 cup freekeh (could also use quinoa or farro)
- [ ] Currants (need 1 cup)
- [ ] Chickpea flour (need ¾ cup)
- [ ] Baking soda

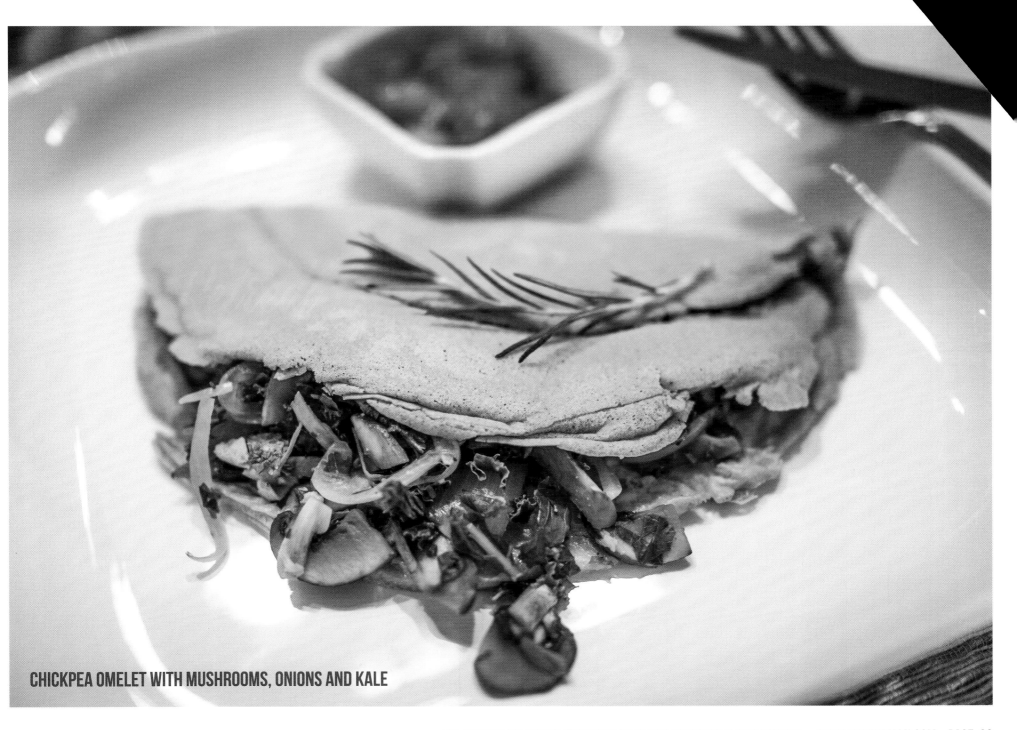

CHICKPEA OMELET WITH MUSHROOMS, ONIONS AND KALE

DAY 11

The diet-style of most Americans is extremely unhealthy. The result is that almost all Americans develop heart disease, regardless of genetics. Autopsy studies on adult Americans of all ages who die in car accidents show that more than 90 percent of them have some degree of atherosclerotic heart disease.

BREAKFAST

CHICKPEA OMELET WITH MUSHROOMS, ONIONS AND KALE
2 SERVINGS

For the Omelet Batter:
¾ cup chickpea flour
½ cup unsweetened soy, hemp or almond milk plus more if needed
2 teaspoons apple cider vinegar
2 teaspoons nutritional yeast
½ teaspoon Dr. Fuhrman's MatoZest (or other no-salt seasoning blend, adjusted to taste)
½ teaspoon ground turmeric
¼ teaspoon baking soda
⅛ teaspoon black pepper

For the Vegetables:
½ cup chopped onions
½ cup chopped red pepper
2 cloves garlic, chopped
1 cup sliced mushrooms
2 cups thinly sliced kale
½ cup low sodium salsa or chopped tomato (see note)

In a small bowl, whisk together the omelet batter ingredients. Add an additional 1-2 tablespoons of non-dairy milk if mixture is too thick to pour.

In a 10-inch, non-stick skillet, heat 2-3 tablespoons water and sauté onions, red pepper and garlic for 2 minutes, add mushrooms and continue to cook until soft and tender, about 3 more minutes. Add kale and stir until wilted. Remove from pan.

Clean skillet and lightly wipe with olive oil. Pour half of the batter into the pan and swirl to evenly cover the bottom. Place half of the sautéed vegetables on top of one side of the omelet. Cook until the omelet bubbles and starts to firm up along the edges (about 2 minutes).

Gently fold over one side and cook for another minute. Cover with a lid, remove from heat and allow to steam for 5 minutes. Repeat to make second omelet. Serve with salsa or chopped tomato.

Note: To make your own salsa, mix together 2 chopped tomatoes, 1 small chopped red onion, 1 clove minced garlic, ½ chopped jalapeño, 3 tablespoons cilantro and 3 tablespoons lime juice.

LUNCH

Green Salad or Raw Veggies with Easy Avocado Dressing (or other leftover dressing)

Include mixed baby greens, shredded red cabbage, tomatoes and red onion in your salad.

EASY AVOCADO DRESSING
SERVES: 4
2 avocados, peeled
1 lime, juiced
1 clove garlic, minced
¼ cup minced onion
2 tablespoons nutritional yeast
⅛ teaspoon cayenne pepper or more to taste
¼ cup water

Blend all ingredients in a high-powered blender until smooth. Add additional water if needed to adjust consistency.

Leftover dressing can be used at dinner tomorrow night.

PORTOBELLO PIZZA
1 SERVING
2 large Portobello mushrooms, stems removed
¼ teaspoon garlic powder
¼ teaspoon dried basil
¼ teaspoon dried oregano
½ cup low-sodium pasta sauce
⅓ cup thinly sliced onion
⅓ cup thinly sliced green or red bell pepper
2-3 tablespoons Nutritarian Parmesan (see note)

Preheat oven to 350 degrees F. Place mushrooms on a parchment-lined baking sheet, gill side up and sprinkle with garlic powder, basil and oregano. Bake for 6 minutes.

Top with tomato sauce, onions and peppers and a sprinkle of Nutritarian Parmesan. Bake for an additional 20 minutes or until vegetables are tender.

Note: To make Nutritarian Parmesan, place ¼ cup almonds or walnuts and ¼ cup nutritional yeast in a food processor and pulse until the texture of grated Parmesan is achieved. Store in an airtight container and refrigerate.

Apple slices with raw almond or cashew butter

DINNER

SPICY CORN AND RED PEPPER SOUP
4 SERVINGS

8 ears sweet corn, kernels removed (or 4 cups frozen)

4 red bell peppers, diced

1 large onion, finely chopped

2 small red chili peppers, or to taste

2 tablespoons finely chopped cilantro

2 tablespoons arrowroot powder (or corn starch)

4 cups low-sodium or no-salt-added vegetable broth

4 cups water

½ cup raw cashews

¼ cup unhulled hemp seeds

1 cup unsweetened soy, hemp or almond milk

black pepper, to taste

Heat ¼ cup water in a soup pot over medium heat, add the corn kernels, red bell peppers, onion and chili peppers and stir well. Reduce heat and cook covered for 10 minutes or until peppers start to soften, stirring occasionally. Increase the heat to medium, add the cilantro and cook, stirring for 30 seconds or until fragrant. Sprinkle with arrowroot powder and stir for 1 minute. Gradually stir in the vegetable broth and water. Bring to a boil, reduce the heat to low and simmer, covered, for 30 minutes.

While soup simmers, blend the cashews, hemp seeds and non-dairy milk in a high-powered blender.

Working in batches, if necessary, add soup to cashew and milk mixture and blend until smooth and creamy. Return to pot and reheat. Season with black pepper.

Perfect Kale Sauté (see Day 1) or other water-sautéed green leafy vegetable

Fresh or frozen raspberries or blackberries for dessert.

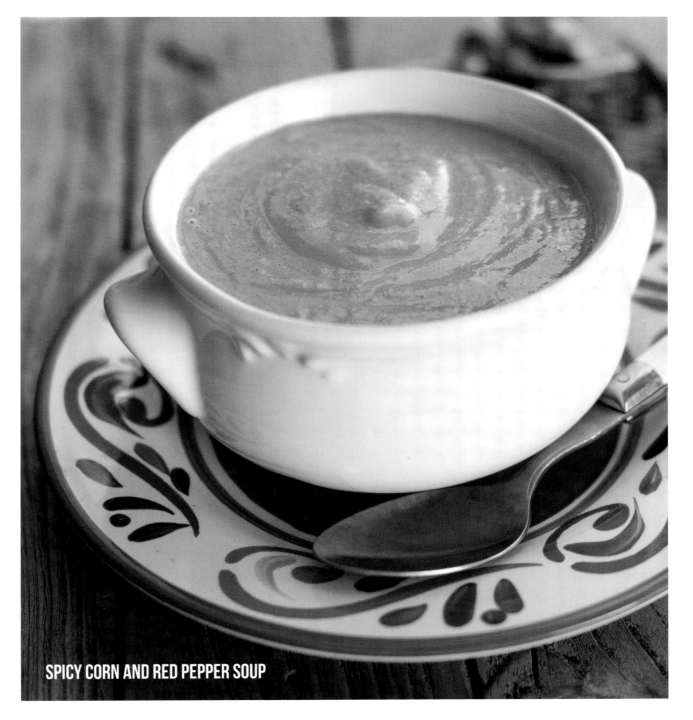

SPICY CORN AND RED PEPPER SOUP

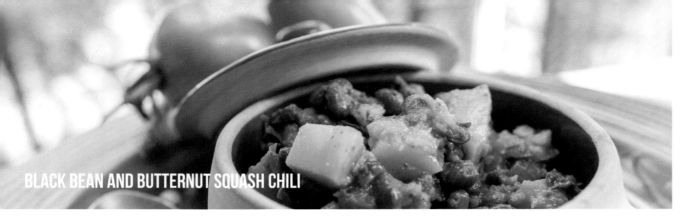

BLACK BEAN AND BUTTERNUT SQUASH CHILI

DAY 12

When a patient with heart disease is not told about effective dietary interventions and instead is offered only drugs, invasive interventional procedures and surgery, than that person is denied informed consent.

BREAKFAST

STRAWBERRY NUT STEEL-CUT OATS
1 SERVING

1 cup water
¼ cup steel-cut oats
½ cup diced apple
1 tablespoon ground flax seeds
½ cup fresh organic or frozen sliced strawberries
2 tablespoons chopped walnuts or pecans

In a saucepan, bring water to a boil and stir in all ingredients, except strawberries and nuts. Reduce heat, cover, and simmer for 15 minutes or until oats are tender and water is absorbed, stirring occasionally.

Stir in strawberries and heat for another minute or two. Remove from heat and stir in nuts.

LUNCH

HUMMUS WRAP
1 SERVING

1 large (100 percent whole grain) tortilla (or large romaine or Swiss chard leaves)
3 tablespoons hummus (see note)
½ cup chopped romaine lettuce
½ cup sliced tomatoes
2 slices red onion
Splash balsamic vinegar

Spread hummus on the wrap or leaves, top with chopped romaine, diced tomatoes, sliced red onion and a splash of balsamic vinegar. Roll up.

Note: To make oil-free, no-salt-added hummus, blend 1 ½ cups cooked chickpeas, 2 tablespoons lemon juice, 2 tablespoons unhulled sesame seeds, 1 garlic clove and ½ teaspoon cumin in a food processor or high-powered blender. Add 1-2 tablespoons water if needed to adjust consistency. (Leftover hummus can be used at lunch tomorrow to make the Hummus Dressing.)

CREAMY CUCUMBER AND ONION SALAD
(or leftover Spicy Corn and Red Pepper Soup from Day 11 dinner)
4 SERVINGS

½ cup unsweetened soy, hemp or almond milk
½ cup raw cashews or ¼ cup raw cashew butter
¼ cup white vinegar
1 teaspoon mustard
1 small clove garlic, peeled
4 large cucumbers, thinly sliced
1 medium white sweet onion, thinly sliced
1 tablespoon fresh dill or 1 teaspoon dried dill

Combine non-dairy milk, cashews, vinegar, mustard and garlic in a high-powered blender and blend until smooth and creamy.

Combine cucumbers, onion and dill and toss with desired amount of dressing. Refrigerate for at least one hour before serving.

Pear or other fresh or frozen fruit for dessert

DINNER

BLACK BEAN AND BUTTERNUT SQUASH CHILI
5 SERVINGS

2 cups chopped onions
3 cloves garlic, chopped
2 ½ cups chopped (½ inch pieces) butternut squash
4 ½ cups cooked or 3 (15 ounce) cans no-salt-added black beans, drained
2 tablespoons chili powder
2 teaspoons ground cumin
2 ½ cups low-sodium or no-salt-added vegetable broth
1 ½ cups no-salt-added diced tomatoes
1 bunch Swiss chard, tough stems removed, chopped

Add all ingredients except Swiss chard to a large pot. Bring to a boil, reduce heat and simmer, uncovered, until squash is tender, about 20 minutes. Stir in Swiss chard and simmer until chard is tender, about 4 minutes longer.

Your choice of a steamed or water-sautéed green vegetable or a salad with leftover Avocado Dressing from Day 11 dinner

Frozen cherries or other fruit for dessert

DAY 13

Refined oils lack the beneficial factors found in whole nuts and seeds. Nuts and seeds contain fiber, minerals, antioxidants and other phytochemicals in addition to healthy fats that contribute to cardiovascular health.

BREAKFAST

BANANA WALNUT BREAKFAST
1 SERVING

1 banana
1 tablespoon ground flax seeds
1 cup blueberries or other berries
¼ cup walnut pieces
¾ cup unsweetened soy, hemp or almond milk

Slice banana into a cereal bowl. Stir in flax seeds, blueberries, walnut pieces, and non-dairy milk.

LUNCH

BIG GREEN SALAD WITH HUMMUS DRESSING

Include romaine lettuce, spinach, tomatoes, radishes and walnuts in your salad.

To make Hummus Dressing, whisk together 3 tablespoons low-sodium hummus (can use leftover hummus from Day 12 lunch), 1 tablespoon raw almond butter, 1 tablespoon lemon juice and 1 tablespoon water.

Roasted Cauliflower (or leftover Black Bean and Butternut Chili from Day 12 dinner)

Melon or other fruit for dessert

> **Tip:** Tomatoes are a rich source of lycopene, a carotenoid pigment linked to reduced risk of heart disease, cancer and age-related eye disorders.

DINNER

SPICY CHICKPEAS WITH SPINACH
3 SERVINGS

1 medium onion, thinly sliced
1 garlic clove, crushed
2 medium tomatoes, chopped
1-2 green chilies, minced
1 tablespoon ground cumin
1 tablespoon coriander
12 ounces spinach, chopped (frozen or fresh)
2 cups cooked chickpeas or 1 (15 ounce) can no-salt-added or low-sodium chickpeas, drained
¼ teaspoon cayenne pepper, or to taste

Water sauté onion and garlic until tender. Add the tomatoes, green chilies, cumin, coriander, and spinach. Cook for 5 minutes. Stir in the chickpeas and cayenne pepper and cook for another 5 minutes.

Quinoa (1 cup per serving)
2 clementines or other fresh or frozen fruit

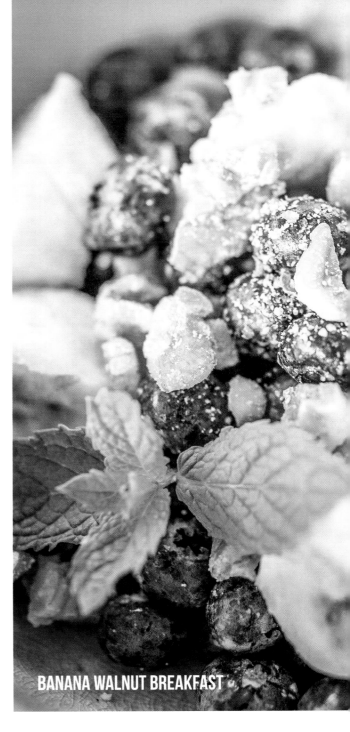

BANANA WALNUT BREAKFAST

DAY 14

The flavonoids in berries, cherries and pomegranates appear to act in several different ways to maintain heart health. These include reducing inflammation, improving blood sugar and lipid levels, lowering blood pressure and preventing plaque formation.

LUNCH

CHERRY SMOOTHIE
2 SERVINGS

2 cups kale, tough stems removed
⅓ cup unsweetened soy, hemp or almond milk
⅓ cup pomegranate juice
⅓ cup carrot juice
1 cup frozen cherries
½ banana
1 tablespoon ground flax seeds

Blend ingredients in a high-powered blender.

Tip: Smoothies are portable and require minimal time and effort to make. They are a great choice for on-the-go breakfasts. Blending fruits and raw, leafy vegetables makes it easier for the body to absorb the beneficial phytochemicals inside each plant's cells.

LUNCH

ANCIENT GRAIN SALAD (SERVE ON A BED OF SHREDDED LETTUCE)
4 SERVINGS

1 cup freekeh (or quinoa or farro)
2 ½ cups water
1 cup shelled edamame (see note)
½ cup diced red bell pepper
¼ cup chopped red onion
¼ cup raisins or currants
1 lime, juiced
2 tablespoons balsamic vinegar
½ cup pineapple, diced
2 tablespoons chopped walnuts

In a medium saucepan, combine the freekeh and water, bring to a boil. Reduce heat to low, cover and simmer for 20-25 minutes or until freekeh is tender and water has been absorbed. Let cool.

Transfer freekeh to a mixing bowl and stir in remaining ingredients. Chill before serving.

Note: Cooked green peas or other varieties of cooked beans may be substituted for the edamame.

BAKED EGGPLANT

Prick the eggplant with a fork in several places. Bake for 45-60 minutes or until tender at 300 degrees F. Slice in half, mash and if desired, sprinkle with cinnamon. Top with water-sautéed onions.

Melon or other fruit for dessert

DINNER

Raw Veggies with Easy Avocado Dressing (see Day 11)

SPAGHETTI SQUASH PRIMAVERA
4 SERVINGS

1 medium spaghetti squash
1 ½ carrots, sliced
½ cup sliced celery
3 cloves garlic, minced
1 ½ cups shredded cabbage
1 small zucchini, chopped into small pieces
1 ½ cups cooked or 1 (15 ounce) can no-salt-added pinto beans, drained
1 ½ cups chopped tomatoes
⅓ cup no-salt-added vegetable broth
1 teaspoon dried thyme
1 tablespoon fresh parsley
½ teaspoon crushed red pepper
1 teaspoon ground coriander
1 cup no-salt-added or low-sodium pasta sauce

Preheat oven to 350 degrees F. Slice spaghetti squash in half lengthwise; remove seeds. Place both halves upside down on a baking sheet. Bake for 45 minutes or until tender.

Meanwhile, cook carrots and celery in 2 tablespoons of water in a covered pan over medium heat for 5 minutes, stirring occasionally, adding a little more water if needed. Add garlic, cabbage, and zucchini and cook, covered, for another 10 minutes. Stir in remaining ingredients, except for pasta sauce. Cover and simmer for 10 minutes or until vegetables are tender.

When the squash is done, remove from oven and using a fork, scrape spaghetti-like strands from squash into a bowl. Stir in the pasta sauce, then combine with the vegetable and bean mixture.

Note: Can be topped with a sprinkle of Nutritarian Parmesan. (See Day 11 lunch)

Tip: Walnuts, hemp seeds, chia seeds and flaxseeds have the most favorable omega-3 content of all nuts and seeds.

CHIA COOKIES (AND BLACKBERRIES OR RASPBERRIES)

12 SERVINGS

1 cup currants
2 cups finely ground rolled oats
½ cup dried, unsweetened, shredded coconut
1 tablespoon ground chia seeds
1 tablespoon whole chia seeds
1 teaspoon cinnamon
1 apple, peeled and quartered
2 tablespoons raw almond butter
1 teaspoon alcohol-free vanilla flavor

Preheat oven to 200 degrees F. Soak ½ cup of the currants in ½ cup water for at least 1 hour.

Combine the ground oats, coconut, remaining currants, chia seeds and cinnamon in a bowl. Place the apple in a food processor and puree until smooth. Add the almond butter, soaked currants and their soaking water and vanilla. Blend until smooth, then add to the dry ingredients and mix well.

Form cookies using 2 teaspoons of dough per cookie. Place on a baking sheet lightly wiped with oil or covered with parchment paper. Bake at very low heat, 200 degrees F for 1 ½ to 2 hours.

Makes 36 cookies. Serving size is 3 cookies. Leftover cookies can be enjoyed for dessert over the next few days.

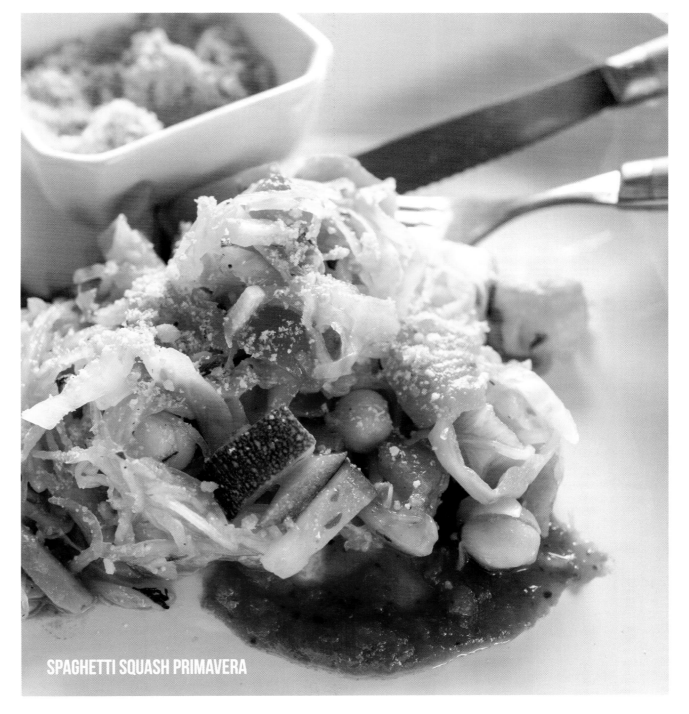

SPAGHETTI SQUASH PRIMAVERA

DAY 15

True protection from heart disease can be reached only when you achieve favorable blood pressure and cholesterol levels without drugs.

BREAKFAST

CAULIFLOWER AND TOFU BENEDICT
2 SERVINGS

4 ounces extra-firm tofu, sliced
½ teaspoon onion powder
½ teaspoon garlic powder
½ head cauliflower, broken into pieces
¼ cup nutritional yeast
½ tablespoon whole wheat flour
½ cup water
¼ cup walnuts, toasted and ground
½ teaspoon Bragg Liquid Aminos or low-sodium soy sauce
1 teaspoon Dijon mustard
¼ teaspoon tarragon
1 large tomatoes, sliced
2 pitas or 2 slices bread (100 percent whole grain),
   lightly toasted
dash paprika
black pepper, to taste

Preheat oven to 325 degrees F. Place sliced tofu on wire rack, sprinkle with garlic and onion powder and bake for 30 minutes or until golden and firm on the outside.

Steam cauliflower for 10-12 minutes or until tender.

To prepare sauce, whisk together nutritional yeast and flour in a small saucepan. Add water, ground walnuts and Bragg Liquid Aminos and stir over medium heat until sauce starts to thicken. Stir in mustard and tarragon.

On each pita or slice of bread, place baked tofu, tomato slices, and steamed cauliflower. Top with sauce. Sprinkle with paprika and black pepper. For a gluten-free option, serve without the bread.

Fresh or frozen blueberries

Tip: Always choose 100 percent whole grain breads and wraps. Look for bread products that are made from intact sprouted grains or coarsely ground grain.

LUNCH

CARIBBEAN BLACK BEAN SALAD
2 SERVINGS

1 ½ cups cooked or 1 (15 ounce) can low-sodium
   black beans, drained
½ cucumber, chopped
1 medium tomato, chopped
2 scallions, thinly sliced
½ cup fresh or thawed frozen corn
½ lime, juiced
¼ cup chopped cilantro,
1 clove garlic, chopped
1-2 tablespoons rice vinegar, to taste
1 teaspoon Dr. Fuhrman's MatoZest (or other no-salt
   seasoning blend, adjusted to taste)

In a large bowl, combine black beans, cucumber, tomato, scallions and corn.

Whisk together remaining ingredients. Toss dressing with black bean mixture.

Steamed Broccoli or other fresh or frozen green vegetable

Pineapple or other fruit for dessert with leftover Chia Cookies from Day 14 dinner

DINNER

MARGARITA COOLER
2 SERVINGS

2 cups green grapes
½ lime, peeled
1 orange, peeled
3 cups kale, large stems removed

Blend ingredients in a high-powered blender until smooth. Pour over ice.

ROASTED VEGETABLE SALAD TOPPED WITH SALMON OR SHIITAKE BACON
2 SERVINGS

1 red pepper, cut into ½ inch pieces
1 small eggplant, cut into ½ inch pieces
1 small yellow squash, cut into ½ inch pieces
1 ½ cups butternut squash, peeled and cut into ½ inch pieces
1 teaspoon olive oil
2 tablespoons balsamic vinegar
3 cloves garlic, minced
1 teaspoon Bragg Liquid Aminos or low-sodium soy sauce
black pepper, to taste
4 ounces wild-caught salmon (or Shiitake Bacon)
⅛ teaspoon garlic powder
8 cups mixed greens

Preheat oven to 400 degrees F. Lightly coat a large baking pan using a paper towel moistened with olive oil. Place vegetables in pan. In a small bowl, combine olive oil, vinegar, garlic, Bragg Liquid Aminos, and black pepper and toss with vegetables. Roast in oven for 18-20 minutes, until tender, stirring once.

Cut salmon into 2 pieces. Season with garlic powder and black pepper. Place salmon, skin side down on a non-stick baking sheet. Bake at 400 degrees F until salmon is cooked through, about 10 minutes. (See recipe below if substituting Shiitake Bacon for salmon.)

Place mixed greens on serving plates. Top with roasted vegetables and salmon or Shiitake Bacon.

SHIITAKE BACON
2 SERVINGS

4 regular or 2 Medjool dates, pitted
1 teaspoon Bragg Liquid Aminos or reduced-sodium soy sauce
1 teaspoon garlic powder
½ teaspoon chili powder
¼ teaspoon ground cumin
¼ cup water
7 ounces shiitake mushroom tops, thinly sliced

Mash together dates, Bragg Liquid Aminos, garlic powder, chili powder, cumin and water in a medium bowl. Add the sliced mushrooms and toss until mushrooms are well coated with date mixture. Spread evenly on a baking sheet lined with parchment paper. Bake at 300 degrees F until mushrooms are dried and browned, about one hour.

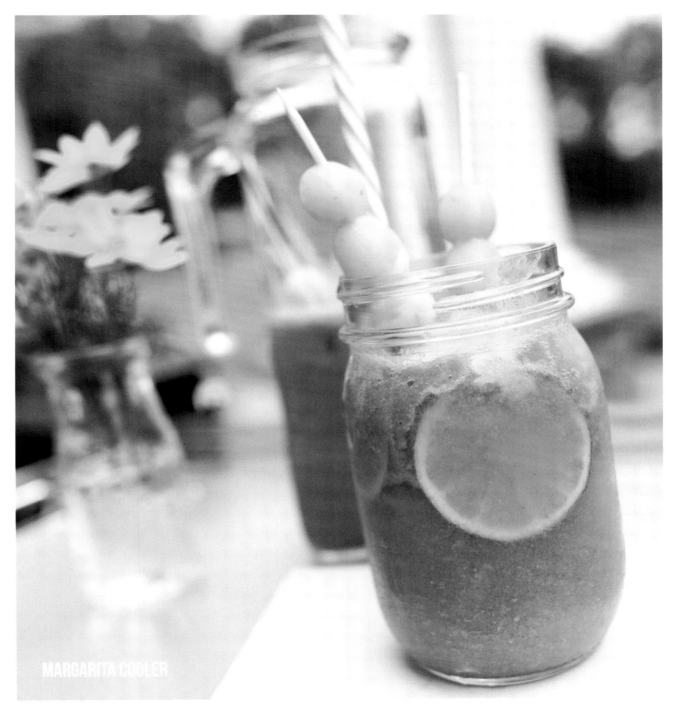

MARGARITA COOLER

DAYS 16-20
SHOPPING LIST

This shopping list assumes that all recipes in the meal plan will be made. Menus frequently include fruit for dessert and will mention a specific fruit as an example. That fruit is used for the shopping list.

Check your refrigerator, freezer and pantry before shopping. You may have items leftover from Days 1-15 that you can use. Make sure you also have all the items listed in the Stock Your Pantry list.

FRESH PRODUCE
VEGETABLES

- [ ] 1 head romaine lettuce
- [ ] 1 head red leaf lettuce
- [ ] Mixed greens (need 5 cups)
- [ ] 2 bunches kale
- [ ] Spinach (need 2 cups)
- [ ] 1 bunch collard greens
- [ ] Green cabbage (need at least ½ head)
- [ ] Red cabbage (need 2 cups)
- [ ] 1 head broccoli
- [ ] Cauliflower (need 1 head plus ¼ head)
- [ ] 1 bunch asparagus
- [ ] Your choice of green leafy vegetable to equal 2 cups cooked (could also buy frozen)
- [ ] Your choice green or high-nutrient non-green vegetable (tomatoes, onions, mushrooms, cauliflower, eggplant and red peppers) to equal 2 cups cooked (could also buy frozen)
- [ ] 4 zucchini
- [ ] 1 cucumber
- [ ] 1 red or green bell pepper

- [ ] 1 jalapeno pepper
- [ ] 1 Anaheim or poblano pepper
- [ ] Carrots (need about 4)
- [ ] Celery (need 4-5 stalks)
- [ ] 6 sweet potatoes
- [ ] 2 avocados
- [ ] 4 tomatoes
- [ ] 1 cup grape or cherry tomatoes
- [ ] 10 ounces white or cremini mushrooms
- [ ] 4 yellow onions
- [ ] 2 red onions
- [ ] Scallions (need 2-3)
- [ ] Radishes (need 2)
- [ ] 3-inch piece of ginger
- [ ] Head of garlic
- [ ] Basil
- [ ] Cilantro

FRUIT

- [ ] 4 cups blueberries (could also use frozen)
- [ ] Small bunch of grapes
- [ ] 2 oranges

- [ ] 2 clementines
- [ ] 6 apples
- [ ] 2 mangos (could also use 3 cups frozen)
- [ ] 3 peaches or nectarines (could also use 3 cups frozen peaches)
- [ ] 2 kiwi
- [ ] 2 bananas
- [ ] 2 lemons
- [ ] 2 limes

REFRIGERATED

- [ ] 3 cups unsweetened, unflavored soy, hemp or almond milk
- [ ] ½ cup carrot juice

FROZEN

This list does not include vegetables and fruit listed under fresh produce list that have a frozen option.

- [ ] Blueberries (need ½ cup)
- [ ] Corn kernels (need 1 ½ cups)

SHELF STABLE
BEANS

It is assumed that except for split peas, canned beans will be used. Select no-salt-added varieties. If you opt to start with dry beans, 1 cup of dry beans will yield about 3 cups of cooked beans.

- [ ] 2 (15 ounce) cans red kidney beans
- [ ] 2 (15 ounce) cans black beans
- [ ] 2 (15 ounce) cans white beans
- [ ] 1 (15 ounce) can no-salt-added chickpeas
- [ ] 1 ¾ cups dried split peas

OTHER

Choose tomato products packaged in BPA-free materials.

- [ ] 4 cups no-salt-added vegetable broth
- [ ] No-salt-added diced tomatoes (need 3 cups)
- [ ] No-salt-added tomato sauce (need 1 cup)
- [ ] Low-sodium tomato juice (3 cups)
- [ ] 2 cups buckwheat groats
- [ ] Corn tortillas
- [ ] Coconut water (need about ½ cup)
- [ ] Dried sage
- [ ] Celery seed
- [ ] Chipotle chili powder (purchased for Days 6-10?)
- [ ] Low-sodium miso paste (purchased for Days 6-10?)

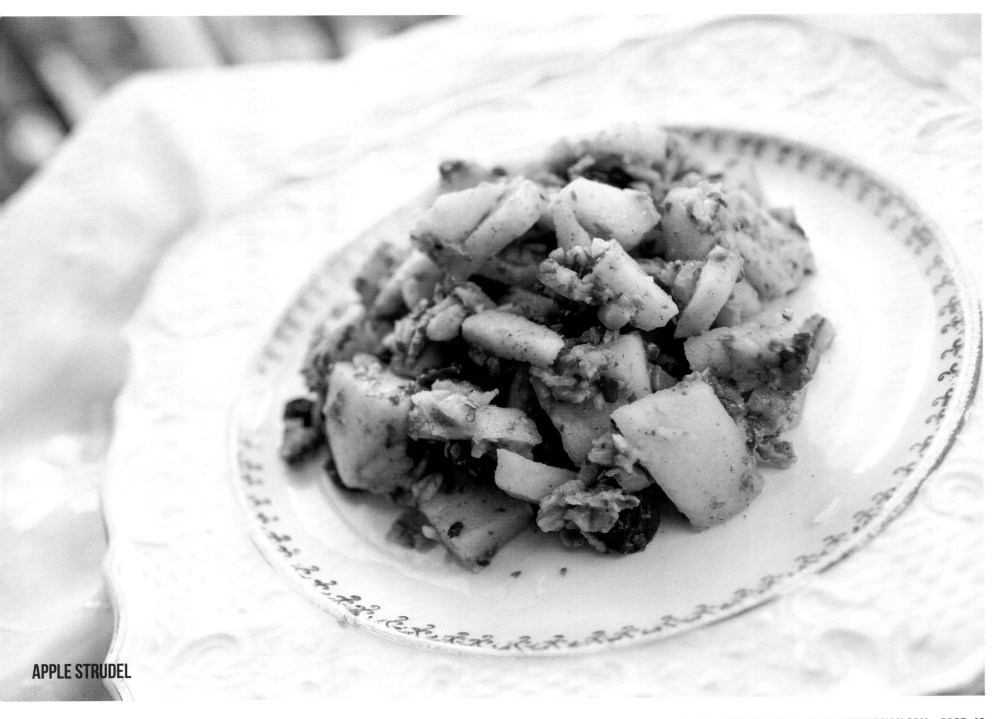

APPLE STRUDEL

DAY 16

The Allium genus of vegetables—onions, garlic, leeks, chives, shallots and scallions—does more than just add great flavor to meals. These vegetables are anti-diabetic, anti-cancer and have beneficial effects on the cardiovascular and immune systems.

BREAKFAST

APPLE STRUDEL
3 SERVINGS

½ cup unsweetened soy, hemp or almond milk
¾ teaspoon alcohol-free vanilla extract or pure vanilla bean powder
1 teaspoon cinnamon
3 apples, peeled, cored and chopped
¼ cup raisins, chopped
½ cup old-fashioned rolled oats
¼ cup ground raw walnuts
2 tablespoons ground flax seeds

Preheat oven to 350 degrees F. In a bowl, mix the non-dairy milk, vanilla and cinnamon until combined. Stir in the chopped apples, raisins, oats, ground walnuts and flax seeds.

Pour into an 8X8 inch baking dish. Bake, uncovered, for 1 hour.

You can have leftover Apple Strudel as an alternative breakfast or even a dessert over the next few days.

LUNCH

CHICKPEA COLLARD WRAPS
3 SERVINGS

1 ½ cups cooked or 1 (15 ounce) can no-salt-added chickpeas, drained
½ cup walnuts
1 teaspoon Bragg Liquid Aminos or low-sodium soy sauce
2 teaspoons lemon juice

1 teaspoon Dr. Fuhrman's MatoZest (or other no-salt seasoning blend adjusted to taste)
6 collard green leaves (see note)
1 cup shredded carrots
1 cup shredded red or green cabbage
¼ cup chopped red onion
1 avocado, peeled and diced

In a food processor, pulse the chickpeas, walnuts, Bragg, lemon juice and no-salt seasoning until crumbled and similar in consistency to ground meat.

Use a paring knife to shave down the thick stalk of the collard leaves to make them easier to roll. Place an equal amount of the chickpea and walnut mixture on each leaf and top with the carrots, cabbage, onion and avocado. Fold up like a burrito.

If desired, serve with a leftover salad dressing or a purchased low-sodium, no-oil dressing.

Note: 100 percent whole grain tortillas can be substituted for the collard leaves

> **Tip:** If you are pressed for time and opt for a bottled salad dressing, use a no-oil dressing that contains no more than 75 mg of sodium per tablespoon.

TOMATO SALAD

Mix together chopped tomatoes, chopped cucumbers, chopped red onion and basil leaves. Sprinkle with balsamic vinegar and season with oregano and black pepper.

BERRY YOGURT
2 SERVINGS

2 cups fresh or frozen blueberries, blackberries or strawberries
¾ cup unsweetened soy, almond or hemp milk
2 tablespoons ground flax or chia seeds
4 regular dates or 2 Medjool dates, pitted

Place ingredients in a high-powered blender and blend until smooth. Chill before serving.

DINNER

GREEN SALAD WITH CURRIED PEANUT BUTTER DRESSING

Include romaine, red leaf lettuce, shredded kale, tomatoes and scallions in your salad.

To make Curried Peanut Butter Dressing, Whisk together 2 tablespoons natural peanut butter, 1 teaspoon curry powder, ½ teaspoon Bragg Liquid Aminos, 1 teaspoon lime juice, 2 teaspoons rice vinegar and 3 tablespoons warm water. Add more water, if needed, to adjust consistency.

HERBED SPLIT PEA SOUP
4 SERVINGS

1 ¾ cups dried split peas
4 cups low-sodium or no-salt-added vegetable broth
3 cups water
2 cloves garlic, minced
¼ teaspoon dried sage

1 teaspoon dried basil

½ teaspoon dried thyme

1 teaspoon no-salt seasoning blend, such as Mrs. Dash

½ cup diced onion

½ cup sliced carrots

½ cup sliced celery

½ cup chopped sweet potato

4 packed cups chopped kale or spinach

Combine split peas, broth, water, garlic, sage, basil, thyme, and no-salt seasoning. Cover and simmer for 30 minutes, stirring occasionally.

Add onions, carrots, celery, and sweet potato. Cover and simmer for another 30 minutes or until vegetables are tender. If using kale, add during the last 15 minutes of cooking time. If using spinach, add at the end of the cooking time and heat until just wilted.

Tip: Soups are an important part of the Nutritarian diet. It is easy to combine a variety of green leafy vegetables, mushrooms, onions, beans and other healthy ingredients all in one pot. When vegetables are simmered together in a soup, all the nutrients are retained with the liquid and the gentle heat prevents nutrient loss.

Grapes or other fresh or frozen fruit for dessert

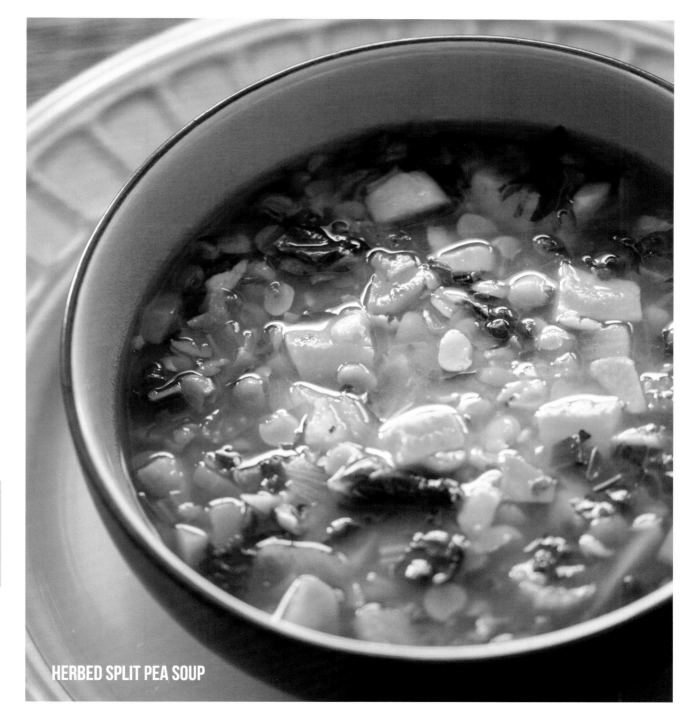

HERBED SPLIT PEA SOUP

DAY 17

If you slip up and have a day where you don't follow the plan, don't get discouraged; just pick up where you left off.

BREAKFAST

BLUEBERRY CHIA SOAKED OATS
(or leftover Apple Strudel from Day 16)

1 SERVING

½ cup old-fashioned oats

1 tablespoon chia seeds

1 cup unsweetened soy, hemp or almond milk

2 tablespoons raisins

½ cup fresh or thawed frozen blueberries (or other fruit)

Combine the oats, chia seeds, non-dairy milk and raisins. Soak for at least 30 minutes or overnight.

Stir in blueberries.

LUNCH

Big green salad with Citrusy Carrot-Ginger Dressing
(or leftover Curried Peanut Butter Dressing from Day 16)

Include in your salad mixed greens, shredded red cabbage, tomatoes and radishes. Top with toasted pumpkin or sunflower seeds.

CITRUSY CARROT-GINGER DRESSING

2 SERVINGS

½ cup carrot juice

1 navel orange, peeled

1 lemon, juiced

¼ cup raw almonds or ⅛ cup raw almond butter

1 inch piece of ginger, peeled

Blend ingredients in a high-powered blender until smooth and creamy.

Steamed Asparagus or other green vegetable
(or Leftover Herbed Split Pea Soup from Day 16)

Fresh or frozen mango or other fruit for dessert

> **Tip:** Nut- and seed-based salad dressings ensure that we get the "good" fats we need, along with their antioxidants, phytochemicals and other health-supporting benefits. The fat from nuts and seeds, when eaten with vegetables, increases the phytochemical absorption from those veggies.

DINNER

SWEET AND SMOKY BAKED BEANS

3 SERVINGS

1 large onion, chopped

4 cloves garlic, chopped

1 cup low-sodium or no-salt-added tomato sauce

1 apple, cored and quartered

¼ cup raisins, soaked in hot water to cover for 30 minutes

1 tablespoon apple cider vinegar

2 tablespoons mustard

1 teaspoon Bragg Liquid Aminos or low-sodium soy sauce

1 teaspoon chipotle chili powder

3 cups cooked or 2 (15 ounce) cans no-salt-added red kidney beans, drained

Preheat oven to 350 degrees F. Heat 2-3 tablespoons water in a small pan and sauté onions and garlic until tender, about 5 minutes. Add small amounts of additional water as needed to prevent burning.

Blend tomato sauce, apple, raisins and soaking water, vinegar, mustard, Bragg Liquid Aminos and chipotle chili powder in a high-powered blender until smooth.

In a large casserole dish, combine the kidney beans, blended mixture and sautéed onions. Cover and bake for 50 minutes.

SHREDDED CABBAGE SLAW

3 SERVINGS

½ medium green cabbage, thinly shredded

1 carrot, shredded

¼ cup finely chopped onion

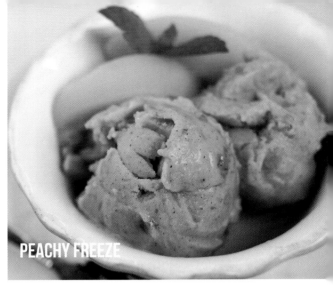

PEACHY FREEZE

1 teaspoon celery seed

⅓ cup raw cashews

1 tablespoon hemp seeds

¼ cup raisins

½ cup unsweetened soy, hemp or almond milk

1 clove garlic

2 tablespoons apple cider vinegar

2 tablespoons lemon juice

1 teaspoon Dijon mustard

In a large bowl, mix together green cabbage, carrot, onion and celery seed. Blend remaining ingredients in a high-powered blender. Toss cabbage mixture with desired amount of dressing.

PEACHY FREEZE

3 SERVINGS

1 ripe banana, frozen

3 ripe peaches or nectarines (peeled and pitted) or 3 cups frozen peaches

4 regular or 2 Medjool dates, pitted

¼ cup unsweetened soy, hemp or almond milk

1 teaspoon alcohol-free vanilla extract or pure vanilla bean powder

⅛ teaspoon cinnamon

Blend ingredients in a high-powered blender until smooth and creamy.

DAY 18

Vitamins, minerals, fiber, antioxidants, bioflavonoids and phytochemicals are all required for normal body function—they are not optional.

BREAKFAST

BLUEBERRY ORANGE SMOOTHIE
1 SERVING

1 orange, peeled and seeded
½ banana
½ cup frozen blueberries
1 tablespoon ground flax seeds
2 cups kale or romaine lettuce

Blend ingredients in a high-powered blender until smooth and creamy.

LUNCH

AVOCADO TOAST WITH SLICED TOMATOES AND TOASTED PUMPKIN SEEDS
1 SERVING

1 (100 percent whole grain) pita, lightly toasted
½ ripe avocado, mashed
1 small tomato, sliced
¼ red onion, sliced thinly
2 tablespoons raw pumpkin seeds, toasted (see note)
black pepper or crushed red pepper flakes, to taste

Spread the mashed avocado on top of the toasted pita. Add tomato slices and sliced onion and sprinkle with pumpkin seeds. Season with your choice of ground black pepper or red pepper flakes.

Note: Other seeds or chopped nuts may be substituted.

Shredded Cabbage Slaw (from Day 17 dinner) or raw veggies with your choice of dressing from another day

2 kiwi or other fruit for dessert

DINNER

LEMON HERB CAULIFLOWER RICE
2 SERVINGS

1 head cauliflower, cut into florets
2 cloves garlic, chopped
2 tablespoons lemon juice
¼ cup chopped fresh basil, dill or parsley
¼ cup chopped almonds and/or raisins

Grate cauliflower or pulse in a food processor until it resembles rice.

Add 2 tablespoons of water and "riced" cauliflower to a skillet. Cover and cook for 8 minutes, add garlic and cook for an additional 2 minutes. Add additional water, if needed, to prevent sticking.

Remove from heat and stir in lemon juice, herbs and chopped almonds and/or raisins.

Steamed or water-sautéed green leafy vegetable such as kale, collards or Swiss chard.

Apple slices with raw almond or cashew butter for dessert

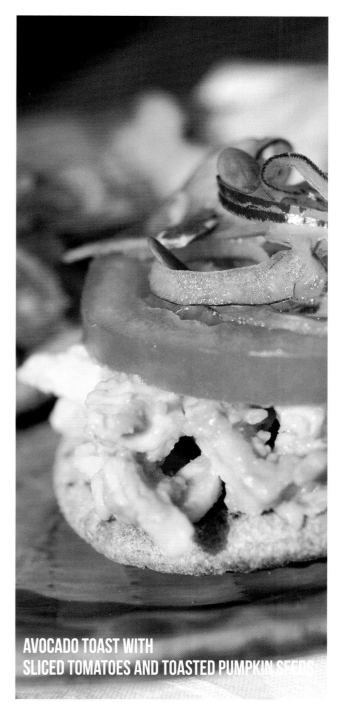

AVOCADO TOAST WITH
SLICED TOMATOES AND TOASTED PUMPKIN SEEDS

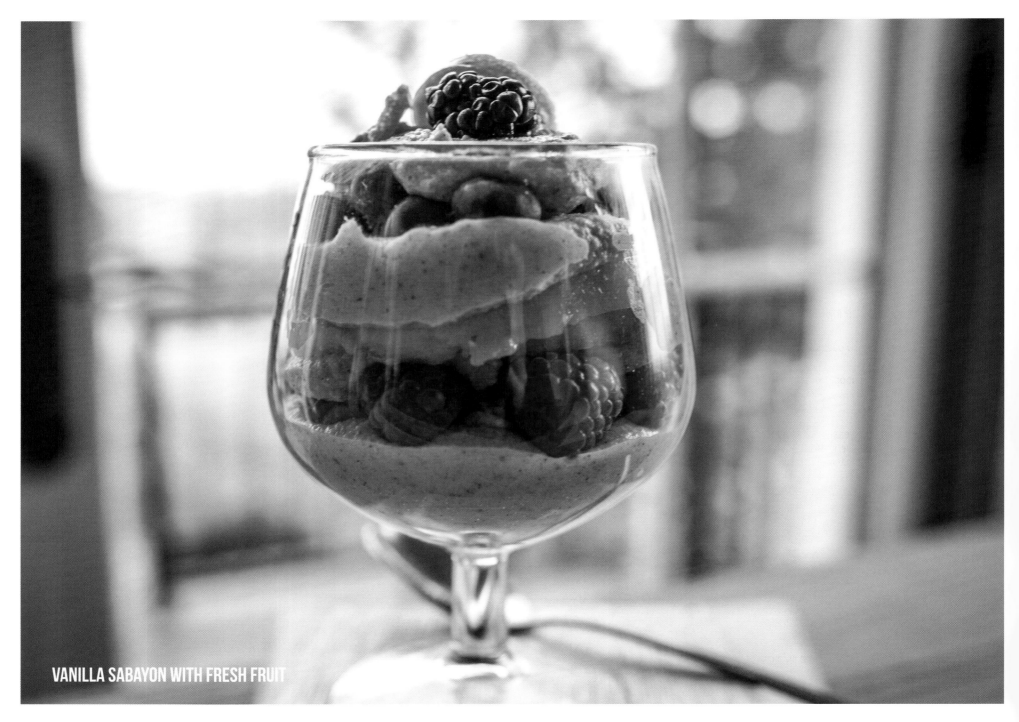

VANILLA SABAYON WITH FRESH FRUIT

DAY 19

In the typical American diet, about 30 percent of calories come from animal foods such as dairy, meat, eggs and chicken, and about 55 percent come from processed foods such as pasta, bread, soda, oils, sugar, puffed cereals, pretzels and other refined products. Cancer and heart disease are the inevitable consequences.

BREAKFAST
SCRAMBLED OATS
3 SERVINGS

1 cup steel-cut oats (see note)
2 cups water (or no-salt-added or low-sodium vegetable broth)
1 tablespoon nutritional yeast
1 teaspoon reduced-sodium miso paste
½ teaspoon ground turmeric
2 cups fresh spinach or other chopped leafy greens
1 cup lightly sautéed sliced mushrooms
grated red or yellow onion for garnish

Combine oats, water, nutritional yeast, miso and turmeric in a saucepan and cook, stirring frequently, for about 20 minutes or until oats are tender. Stir in spinach and mushrooms and cook until spinach is wilted. Garnish with grated onion.

Note: You may also use old-fashioned oats in this recipe. Reduce cooking time to 5 minutes.

Halved cherry or grape tomatoes

LUNCH
TANGY WHITE BEANS AND ZUCCHINI
(serve on a big bed of mixed salad greens)
2 SERVINGS

3 medium zucchini, cut into small chunks
2 cloves garlic, minced

1 ½ cups cooked or 1 (15 ounce) can no-salt-added white beans, drained
¼ cup Dr. Fuhrman's Black Fig Vinegar, other flavored vinegar or balsamic vinegar

Sauté zucchini and garlic in 2 tablespoons water over medium heat for 5 minutes or until tender. Add beans and vinegar and cook for 5 minutes.

Fresh or frozen berries topped with chopped walnuts and shredded coconut for dessert

DINNER
WEST AFRICAN SWEET POTATO SOUP
4 SERVINGS

1 large onion, chopped
1 cup chopped celery
2 tablespoons minced fresh ginger
⅛ teaspoon hot pepper flakes, or to taste
4 cups peeled chopped sweet potatoes
3 cups water
3 cups low-sodium tomato juice
1 cup natural, no-salt-added peanut butter
¼ cup chopped parsley or cilantro

Heat 2-3 tablespoons water in a soup pot and water sauté onions and celery until tender. Stir in the ginger and hot pepper flakes and sauté for one minute. Add sweet potatoes and water, bring to a boil, cover, reduce heat and simmer until potatoes are very tender, about 20 minutes.

Stir in tomato juice and peanut butter. Working in batches, blend the soup in a high-powered blender. Return to the pot, add the parsley or cilantro and reheat.

Steamed or water-sautéed green or other high-nutrient vegetable (can be fresh or frozen)
The high-nutrient, non-green vegetables are: tomatoes, onions, mushrooms, cauliflower, eggplant and red peppers.

VANILLA SABAYON WITH FRESH FRUIT
4 SERVINGS

1 cup raw cashews, soaked overnight
8 regular or 4 Medjool dates, pitted
⅓-½ cup coconut water, as needed
½ teaspoon alcohol-free vanilla extract or pure vanilla bean powder
your choice of fruit

In a high-powered blender, combine all ingredients except for the fruit and blend until very smooth, adding more coconut water as needed to achieve a thick but pourable mixture. Refrigerate. Spoon over fresh fruit.

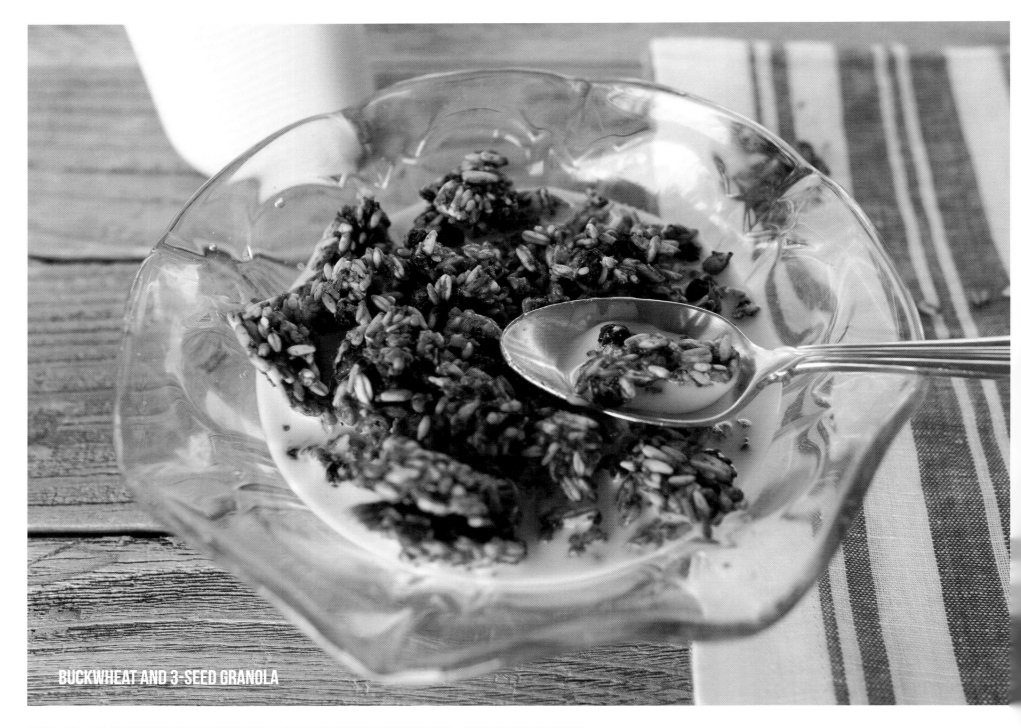

BUCKWHEAT AND 3-SEED GRANOLA

DAY 20

Eating healthfully is the single most effective preventative and therapeutic invention available. It is the best "prescription" any doctor can make.

BREAKFAST

BUCKWHEAT AND 3-SEED GRANOLA (WITH NON-DAIRY MILK AND FRESH OR FROZEN BERRIES)

6 SERVINGS

2 cups raw buckwheat groats (see note)
¼ cup hemp seeds
¼ cup raw sunflower seeds
½ cup currants or raisins
1 cup chopped apple (unpeeled)
½ cup chopped dates, packed tightly
2 tablespoons ground chia seeds
2 teaspoons ground cinnamon
7-8 tablespoons coconut water

Preheat the oven to 300 degrees F. In a large mixing bowl, combine the buckwheat, hemp, sunflower seeds and currants.

Puree the remaining ingredients in a high-powered blender, adding just enough coconut water in tablespoon increments to facilitate blending. Stir the puree into the dry ingredients and coat thoroughly.

Spread on a Silpat-lined baking sheet and bake for 30 minutes, stir and bake for another 20-30 minutes until dry to the touch. It will continue to crisp up as it cools.

Serve with unsweetened non-dairy milk, some berries and banana slices or eat dry, sprinkled on top of fruit.

Note: Buckwheat groats are the gluten-free seeds of the buckwheat plant.

LUNCH

CRUCIFEROUS CRUNCH FULL MEAL SALAD

2 SERVINGS

For the Dressing:
½ cup raw almonds
¼ cup fresh lemon or lime juice
1 tablespoons apple cider vinegar
2 regular or 1 Medjool date, pitted
1 clove garlic
¾ cup water

For the Salad:
½ bunch kale, tough stems removed, torn into small pieces
½ bunch broccoli
¼ head cauliflower
½ small red onion
1 ½ cups cooked or 1 (15 ounce) can no-salt-added white beans, drained
2 tablespoons currants or raisins
¼ cup coarsely chopped walnuts

Blend salad dressing ingredients for 2 minutes until smooth and creamy.

To make the salad: pulse kale, broccoli, cauliflower and onion in a food processor. Place in a large bowl and toss with beans, currants and desired amount of dressing. Serve topped with walnuts.

2 clementines or other fresh or frozen fruit for dessert

DINNER

BEAN ENCHILADA BAKE

10 SERVINGS

1 large onion, chopped
1 Anaheim pepper, chopped
1 jalapeño pepper, chopped
1 red or green bell pepper, chopped
1 large sweet potato, peeled and chopped in small cubes
1 tablespoon ground cumin
2 tablespoons chili powder
3 cups cooked or 2 (15 ounce) cans no-salt-added black beans, drained
3 cups diced tomatoes
1 ½ cups frozen sweet corn kernels
¼ cup chopped fresh cilantro
12 corn tortillas
¼ cup pumpkin seeds
½ cup guacamole and/or low-sodium salsa, optional

Water sauté onions and peppers, add sweet potatoes, spices, beans, tomatoes, frozen corn and cilantro. Simmer for 30 minutes or until potatoes are cooked through. Add a small amount of water if mixture gets too dry.

Lightly wipe a 13"x 9"x 2" baking pan with oil. Place a small amount of chili mixture on bottom, then layer 6 tortillas, chili mixture, remaining tortillas and remaining chili mixture. Sprinkle with pumpkin seeds. Bake at 375 degrees F for 20-30 minutes.

Serve with guacamole and salsa if desired.

Steamed or water-sautéed broccoli or other fresh or frozen green vegetable

Sliced mango or other fruit for dessert

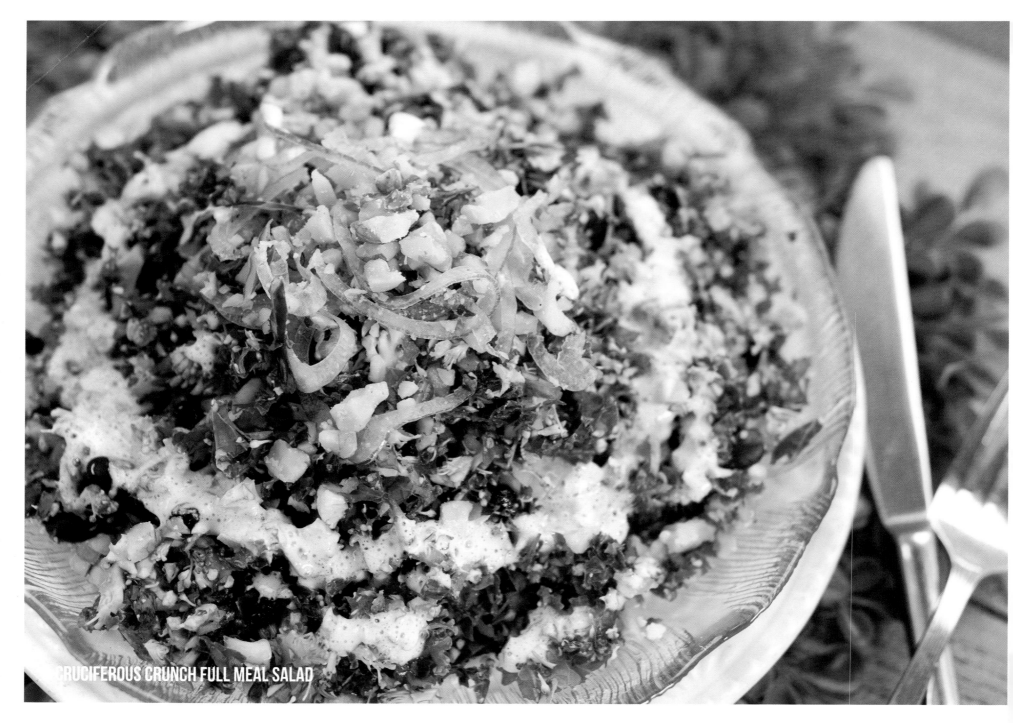

CRUCIFEROUS CRUNCH FULL MEAL SALAD

CONGRATULATIONS!

YOU HAVE COMPLETED DAY 20!

Congratulations on completing Day 20 of the *Transformation 20 Blood Pressure and Cholesterol* Program!

By now, if you have faithfully adhered to the program, you have undoubtedly made great progress in your quest to lower your blood pressure and cholesterol levels. As part of that process, I trust you have been able to reduce or eliminate your medication.

I hope you are encouraged by the improvements you have made to your health and that you would like to see even more. **Don't stop now.** Use your current results as momentum to push yourself forward to make even more progress.

You can, and should, make these changes permanent.
Repeat the menus for one or more additional 20-day cycles, or log onto *DrFuhrman.com* to try our other exciting recipes. You can also design your own menus based on my Nutritarian principles.

Help is always available in navigating the road to better health. Find out more about the Nutritarian eating style, get cooking advice and learn other compelling reasons to adopt this type of diet by reading one or more of my books and utilizing the resources found on my website, *DrFuhrman.com*.

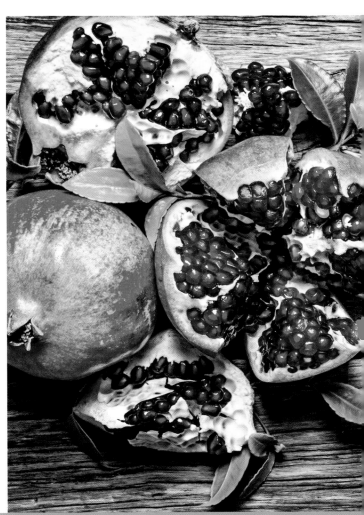

WHAT'S NEXT?

LEARN

Now that you are familiar with how the Nutritarian eating style works, find out more about why it works. The next step on your wellness journey is to read one or more of my *New York Times* best-selling books: *Eat to Live, The End of Dieting, The End of Heart Disease* or *The End of Diabetes*. For parents, there is *Disease-Proof Your Child* and all should read his recent eye-opening work, *Fast Food Genocide*.

These books will give you the in-depth knowledge and practical tools you need to make the Nutritarian eating style your way of life. You'll learn how eating a nutrient-dense, plant-rich diet is a powerful tool for achieving sustainable weight loss and for preventing and reversing chronic diseases, such as heart disease, diabetes, cancer, migraines and autoimmune diseases.
https://shop.drfuhrman.com/books-video

JOIN

Support is a key factor in helping you reach your health and weight loss goals. Membership at DrFuhrman.com gives you that support. You will have access to:

- Nutritarian Recipe database with 1,700+ recipes
- Meal Plans you can download
- Monthly Nutri-Talk / Q&A with Dr. Fuhrman
- Dr. Fuhrman's Video-on-Demand Library

- Position Papers library (download)
- Nutritarian Network online forum
- Living Nutritarian e-magazine (download)
- Connect with Dr. Fuhrman and Dr. Benson in the Ask the Doctor forum**
- Exclusive member promotions

There's a membership level to suit every budget – and you can choose from monthly, annual or lifetime plans.
https://www.drfuhrman.com/membership

* Platinum and Diamond members can post questions in the Ask the Doctor forum. Gold members can view questions and discussions.

GROW

Sometimes, we need extra support when making the transition to the Nutritarian eating style. Dr. Fuhrman's Success Program's licensed clinicians will show you how to put an end to emotional eating, binges, cravings, and other addictive food behaviors. Get the help you need to ensure SUCCESS!

No more addictive food cravings, yo-yo dieting, or emotional eating. Your counselor will:

- Guide you through the foundation of the Nutritarian diet – because knowledge trumps willpower

- Create an action plan based on your unique needs
- Show you how to take action "right now" to make immediate changes in your life
- Review your food diary daily to hold you accountable

Connect with your counselor either in-person at our office, by phone or online – whatever is most convenient for you. Discuss your challenges and gain strategizes for your success! For more information, call our medical practice at (908) 237-0200 or visit
https://www.drfuhrman.com/medical-practice/food-addiction-program

EXPLORE

Support your healthy lifestyle by choosing supplements and food products that are free of problematic ingredients. You can also browse our stock of books, videos and kitchen items. Visit the Shop at DrFuhrman.com for:

- Multivitamins and supplements
- Gourmet foods (soups, dressings, vinegars, Nutrition bars and more)
- *New York Times* best-sellers (print, digital and audio titles)

Also, be sure to check the E-Learning section for updates on Dr. Fuhrman's Guided Detox programs (which take place a few times each year), the Personalized Vitamin Advisor, and the Events section for upcoming U.S. and international vacation getaways with Dr. Fuhrman and his wife, Lisa.

DR. FUHRMAN'S
ADDITIONAL SERVICES

DR. FUHRMAN'S MEDICAL PRACTICE

www.drfuhrman.com/medical-practice
Call for an appointment: (908) 237-0200
Specializing in nutritional and natural medicine to prevent and reverse chronic disease, boost immunity, slow aging and achieve ideal weight and superior health.

In-Office and Remote appointments available.
We offer **Comprehensive medical appointments** (1 hour) and **Condensed medical appointments** (15 minutes). Please note: Condensed medical appointments are scheduled at the sole discretion of the medical office; patients with multiple health issues or complicated diagnoses will be referred to the hour-long comprehensive medical appointment.

Remote consultations available in: California, Florida, Georgia, Illinois, New York, North Carolina, Ohio, Pennsylvania, Texas, Tennessee and Washington

DR. FUHRMAN'S SUCCESS PROGRAM

www.drfuhrman.com/medical-practice/food-addiction-program
Call us today at (908) 237-0200 to find out more.
Put an end to emotional eating, binges, cravings, and other addictive food behaviors with this supportive program.

Our licensed counselor will guide you through the foundation of the Nutritarian diet, create an action plan based on your needs, and review your food diary daily to hold you accountable. Members can take part in a monthly online group chat session.

DR. FUHRMAN'S NUTRITARIAN EDUCATION INSTITUTE

www.drfuhrman.com/nei
Take one course or two and become an expert in the nutrient-dense, plant-rich eating style. Dr. Fuhrman's Nutritarian Studies Program is an online certificate program that teaches the basics of nutrition and the scientific principles behind the Nutritarian eating style. The Art of Nutritarian Cooking certifies you as a Nutritarian chef. The courses are self-paced and structured, with guided lesson plans. * Successful completion of each course may qualify for Continuing Education Unit (CEU) credits.

* Successful completion of each course may qualify for Continuing Education Unit (CEU) credits.

DR. FUHRMAN'S PRODUCTS

https://shop.drfuhrman.com
Browse Dr. Fuhrman's products in the online shop. You'll discover multivitamins for men, women and children; high-quality supplements made from whole-food extracts; food products made without salt, oil, sweeteners or other potentially harmful ingredients; books and media, and much more.

DR. FUHRMAN DESTINATION EVENTS

Enjoy a luxury vacation and health getaway
www.drfuhrman.com/events
Join Dr. Fuhrman and his wife, Lisa, for an unforgettable vacation experience at destinations across the United States and Europe. You'll spend time with Dr. Fuhrman in this relaxed atmosphere, and come back with memories – and important nutritional knowledge – that will last a lifetime. Visit DrFuhrman.com/retreats to view our upcoming events, and make your reservation today.

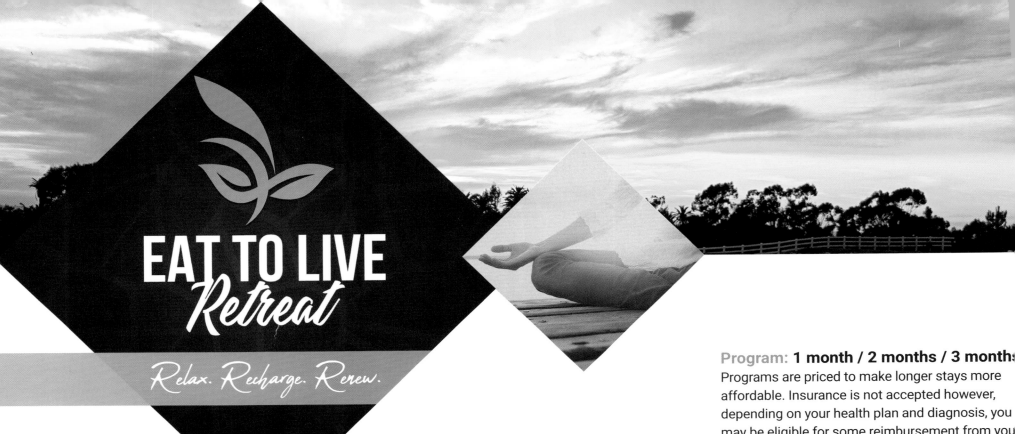

EAT TO LIVE
Retreat

Relax. Recharge. Renew.

Set in San Diego County, California, Dr. Fuhrman's Eat to Live Retreat **is a place of transformation. Come and discover the joy of living in great health.**

For more information or to book your stay, call (949) 432-6295 or email info@ETLRetreat.com www.drfuhrman.com/etlretreat

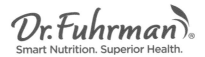

At Dr. Fuhrman's Eat to Live Retreat, you will change your food preferences, resolve your food cravings and addictions, and feel more in control of your health destiny as you embark on your journey to lose excess weight and reverse chronic disease.

The services and products included with each stay are:
- Private guest room with ensuite bathroom
- All organic, plant-based meals
- Entrance & exit consultation with Dr. Fuhrman
- Non-invasive health screenings and consultations with our registered nurse
- Nutrition lectures and education talks
- Cooking classes with our world-class chefs
- Group fitness classes including: circuit training, water aerobics, yoga, meditation, and hiking

Program: 1 month / 2 months / 3 months
Programs are priced to make longer stays more affordable. Insurance is not accepted however, depending on your health plan and diagnosis, you may be eligible for some reimbursement from your insurance company.

About the Eat to Live Retreat
Dr. Fuhrman's Eat to Live Retreat is a unique year-round, residential program where you can transform your health in a profound and lasting way. Under the care and guidance of Dr. Fuhrman and his expert staff, you can achieve dramatic weight loss, recover from chronic disease, reduce or eliminate your need for medications, resolve emotional eating, or simply detox in a supportive environment. The retreat is housed in a stunning property located 30 minutes north of downtown San Diego. The open-air design lends the retreat relaxing atmosphere, where you can reclaim your health in a comfortable environment.

REFERENCES

1. Fuhrman J, Singer M. **Improved cardiovascular parameter with a nutrient-dense, plant-rich diet-style: A patient survey with illustrative cases.** *Am J Lifestyle Med* 2015.

2. Swaminathan RV, Alexander KP. **Pulse pressure and vascular risk in the elderly: associations and clinical implications.** *Am J Geriatr Cardiol* 2006, **15:**226-232; quiz 133-224.

3. Banach M, Aronow WS. **Blood pressure j-curve: current concepts.** *Curr Hypertens Rep* 2012, **14:**556-566.

4. Gupta AK, Dahlof B, Dobson J, et al. **Determinants of new-onset diabetes among 19,257 hypertensive patients randomized in the Anglo-Scandinavian Cardiac Outcomes Trial--Blood Pressure Lowering Arm and the relative influence of antihypertensive medication.** *Diabetes Care* 2008, **31:**982-988.

5. Elliott WJ, Meyer PM. **Incident diabetes in clinical trials of antihypertensive drugs: a network meta-analysis.** *Lancet* 2007, **369:**201-207.

6. Largent JA, Bernstein L, Horn-Ross PL, et al. **Hypertension, antihypertensive medication use, and breast cancer risk in the California Teachers Study cohort.** *Cancer Causes Control* 2010, **21:**1615-1624.

7. Li CI, Daling JR, Tang MT, et al. **Use of antihypertensive medications and breast cancer risk among women aged 55 to 74 years.** *JAMA Intern Med* 2013.

8. U.S. Centers for Disease Control and Prevention: Statin drug use in the past 30 days among adults 45 years of age and over, by sex and age: United States, 1988–1994, 1999–2002, and 2005–2008 [http://www.cdc.gov/nchs/data/hus/2010/fig17.pdf]

9. Sattar N, Preiss D, Murray HM, et al. **Statins and risk of incident diabetes: a collaborative meta-analysis of randomised statin trials.** *Lancet* 2010, **375:**735-742.

10. Rajpathak SN, Kumbhani DJ, Crandall J, et al. **Statin therapy and risk of developing type 2 diabetes: a meta-analysis.** *Diabetes Care* 2009, **32:**1924-1929.

11. Dormuth CR, Hemmelgarn BR, Paterson JM, et al. **Use of high potency statins and rates of admission for acute kidney injury: multicenter, retrospective observational analysis of administrative databases.** *BMJ* 2013, **346:**f880.

12. Okuyama H, Langsjoen PH, Hamazaki T, et al. **Statins stimulate atherosclerosis and heart failure: pharmacological mechanisms.** *Expert Rev Clin Pharmacol* 2015, **8:**189-199.

13. Fuhrman J: *The End of Heart Disease.* New York: HarperCollins; 2016.

14. Bai Y, Wang X, Zhao S, et al. **Sulforaphane Protects against Cardiovascular Disease via Nrf2 Activation.** *Oxid Med Cell Longev* 2015, **2015:**407580.

15. Lidder S, Webb AJ. **Vascular effects of dietary nitrate (as found in green leafy vegetables and beetroot) via the nitrate-nitrite-nitric oxide pathway.** *Br J Clin Pharmacol* 2013, **75:**677-696.

16. Papanikolaou Y, Fulgoni VL, 3rd. **Bean consumption is associated with greater nutrient intake, reduced systolic blood pressure, lower body weight, and a smaller waist circumference in adults: results from the National Health and Nutrition Examination Survey 1999-2002.** *J Am Coll Nutr* 2008, **27:**569-576.

17. Bazzano LA, Thompson AM, Tees MT, et al. **Non-soy legume consumption lowers cholesterol levels: a meta-analysis of randomized controlled trials.** *Nutrition, metabolism, and cardiovascular diseases : NMCD* 2011, **21:**94-103.

18. Streppel MT, Arends LR, van 't Veer P, et al. **Dietary fiber and blood pressure: a meta-analysis of randomized placebo-controlled trials.** *Arch Intern Med* 2005, **165:**150-156.

19. Grosso G, Yang J, Marventano S, et al. **Nut consumption on all-cause, cardiovascular, and cancer mortality risk: a systematic review and meta-analysis of epidemiologic studies.** *Am J Clin Nutr* 2015, **101:**783-793.

20. Del Gobbo LC, Falk MC, Feldman R, et al. **Effects of tree nuts on blood lipids, apolipoproteins, and blood pressure: systematic review, meta-analysis, and dose-response of 61 controlled intervention trials.** *Am J Clin Nutr* 2015, **102:**1347-1356.

21. Kris-Etherton PM, Hu FB, Ros E, Sabate J. **The role of tree nuts and peanuts in the prevention of coronary heart disease: multiple potential mechanisms.** *J Nutr* 2008, **138:**1746S-1751S.

22. Rajaram S, Sabate J. **Nuts, body weight and insulin resistance.** *Br J Nutr* 2006, **96 Suppl 2:**S79-86.

23. Basu A, Rhone M, Lyons TJ. **Berries: emerging impact on cardiovascular health.** *Nutr Rev* 2010, **68:**168-177.

24. Aviram M, Rosenblat M, Gaitini D, et al. **Pomegranate juice consumption for 3 years by patients with carotid artery stenosis reduces common carotid intima-media thickness, blood pressure and LDL oxidation.** *Clin Nutr* 2004, **23:**423-433.

25. Aviram M, Dornfeld L. **Pomegranate juice consumption inhibits serum angiotensin converting enzyme activity and reduces systolic blood pressure.** *Atherosclerosis* 2001, **158:**195-198.

26. Aviram M, Volkova N, Coleman R, et al. **Pomegranate phenolics from the peels, arils, and flowers are antiatherogenic: studies in vivo in atherosclerotic apolipoprotein e-deficient (E 0) mice and in vitro in cultured macrophages and lipoproteins.** *Journal of Agricultural and Food Chemis ry* 2008, **56:**1148-1157.

27. Khalesi S, Irwin C, Schubert M. **Flaxseed consumption may reduce blood pressure: a systematic review and meta-analysis of controlled trials.** *J Nutr* 2015, **145:**758-765.

28. Palozza P, Parrone N, Catalano A, Simone R. **Tomato lycopene and inflammatory cascade: basic interactions and clinical implications.** *Curr Med Chem* 2010, **21:**2547-2563.

29. Karppi J, Laukkanen JA, Sivenius J, et al. **Serum lycopene decreases the risk of stroke in men: A population-based follow-up study.** *Neurology* 2012, **79:**1540-1547.

30. Karppi J, Laukkanen JA, Makikallio TH, Kurl S. **Low serum lycopene and beta-carotene increase risk of acute myocardial infarction in men.** *Eur J Public Health* 2011.

31. Sesso HD, Buring JE, Norkus EP, Gaziano JM. **Plasma lycopene, other carotenoids, and retinol and the risk of cardiovascular disease in women.** *Am J Clin Nutr* 2004, **79:**47-53.

32. Silaste ML, Alfthan G, Aro A, et al. **Tomato juice decreases LDL cholesterol levels and increases LDL resistance to oxidation.** *Br J Nutr* 2007, **98:**1251-1258.

33. Galeone C, Tavani A, Pelucchi C, et al. **Allium vegetable intake and risk of acute myocardial infarction in Italy.** *Eur J Nutr* 2009, **48:**120-123.

34. Rahman K, Lowe GM. **Garlic and cardiovascular disease: a critical review.** *J Nutr* 2006, **136:**736S-740S.

35. Bradley JM, Organ CL, Lefer DJ. **Garlic-derived organic polysulfides and myocardial protection.** *J Nutr* 2016, **146:**403S-409S.

36. Slimestad R, Fossen T, Vagen IM. **Onions: a source of unique dietary flavonoids.** *J Agric Food Chem* 2007, **55:**10067-10080.

37. Makheja AN, Bailey JM. **Antiplatelet constituents of garlic and onion.** *Agents Actions* 1990, **29:**360-363.

38. Powolny A, Singh S. **Multitargeted prevention and therapy of cancer by diallyl trisulfide and related Allium vegetable-derived organosulfur compounds.** *Cancer Lett* 2008, **269:**305-314.

39. Galeone C, Pelucchi C, Levi F, et al. **Onion and garlic use and human cancer.** *Am J Clin Nutr* 2006, **84:**1027-1032.

40. Martin KR. **Both common and specialty mushrooms inhibit adhesion molecule expression and in vitro binding of monocytes to human aortic endothelial cells in a pro-inflammatory environment.** *Nutr J* 2010, **9:**29.

41. Guillamon E, Garcia-Lafuente A, Lozano M, et al. **Edible mushrooms: role in the prevention of cardiovascular diseases.** *Fitoterapia* 2010, **81:**715-723.

42. Poddar KH, Ames M, Hsin-Jen C, et al. **Positive effect of mushrooms substituted for meat on body weight, body composition, and health parameters. A 1-year randomized clinical trial.** *Appetite* 2013, **71:**379-387.

43. Schulzova V, Hajslova J, Peroutka R, et al. **Influence of storage and household processing on the agaritine content of the cultivated Agaricus mushroom.** *Food Addit Contam* 2002, **19:**853-862.

44. Loader J, Montero D, Lorenzen C, et al. **Acute hyperglycemia impairs vascular function in healthy and cardiometabolic diseased subjects: systematic review and meta-analysis.** *Arterioscler Thromb Vasc Biol* 2015, **35:**2060-2072.

45. Fujimoto K, Hozumi T, Watanabe H, et al. **Acute hyperglycemia induced by oral glucose loading suppresses coronary microcirculation on transthoracic Doppler echocardiography in healthy young adults.** *Echocardiography* 2006, **23:**829-834.

46. Ceriello A, Quagliaro L, Piconi L, et al. **Effect of postprandial hypertriglyceridemia and hyperglycemia on circulating adhesion molecules and oxidative stress generation and the possible role of simvastatin treatment.** *Diabetes* 2004, **53:**701-710.

47. Mapanga RF, Essop MF. **Damaging effects of hyperglycemia on cardiovascular function: spotlight on glucose metabolic pathways.** *Am J Physiol Heart Circ Physiol* 2016, **310:**H153-173.

48. Hegab Z, Gibbons S, Neyses L, Mamas MA. **Role of advanced glycation end products in cardiovascular disease.** *World J Cardiol* 2012, **4:**90-102.

49. Fan J, Song Y, Wang Y, et al. **Dietary glycemic index, glycemic load, and risk of coronary heart disease, stroke, and stroke mortality: a systematic review with meta-analysis.** *PLoS One* 2012, **7:**e52182.

50. Pruser KN, Flynn NE. **Acrylamide in health and disease.** *Front Biosci (Schol Ed)* 2011, **3**:41-51.

51. Goldberg T, Cai W, Peppa M, et al. **Advanced glycoxidation end products in commonly consumed foods.** *J Am Diet Assoc* 2004, **104**:1287-1291.

52. Uribarri J, Woodruff S, Goodman S, et al. **Advanced glycation end products in foods and a practical guide to their reduction in the diet.** *J Am Diet Assoc* 2010, **110**:911-916 e912.

53. Lichtenstein AH. **Dietary trans fatty acids and cardiovascular disease risk: past and present.** *Curr Atheroscler Rep* 2014, **16**:433.

54. Engel S, Tholstrup T. **Butter increased total and LDL cholesterol compared with olive oil but resulted in higher HDL cholesterol compared with a habitual diet.** *Am J Clin Nutr* 2015, **102**:309-315.

55. Wang Y, Lin X, Ouyang YY, et al. **Red and processed meat consumption and mortality: dose-response meta-analysis of prospective cohort studies.** *Public Health Nutr* 2016, **19**:893-905.

56. Pan A, Sun Q, Bernstein AM, et al. **Red meat consumption and mortality: results from 2 prospective cohort studies.** *Arch Intern Med* 2012.

57. Sinha R, Cross AJ, Graubard BI, et al. **Meat intake and mortality: a prospective study of over half a million people.** *Arch Intern Med* 2009, **169**:562-571.

58. Song M, Fung TT, Hu FB, et al. **Association of animal and plant protein intake with all-cause and cause-specific mortality.** *JAMA Intern Med* 2016.

59. Abete I, Romaguera D, Vieira AR, et al. **Association between total, processed, red and white meat consumption and all-cause, CVD and IHD mortality: a meta-analysis of cohort studies.** *Br J Nutr* 2014, **112**:762-775.

60. Chen GC, Lv DB, Pang Z, Liu QF. **Red and processed meat consumption and risk of stroke: a meta-analysis of prospective cohort studies.** *Eur J Clin Nutr* 2013, **67**:91-95.

61. Ahluwalia N, Genoux A, Ferrieres J, et al. **Iron status is associated with carotid atherosclerotic plaques in middle-aged adults.** *J Nutr* 2010, **140**:812-816.

62. Brewer GJ. **Iron and copper toxicity in diseases of aging, particularly atherosclerosis and Alzheimer's disease.** *Exp Biol Med* 2007, **232**:323-335.

63. Tzoulaki I, Brown IJ, Chan Q, et al. **Relation of iron and red meat intake to blood pressure: cross sectional epidemiological study.** *BMJ* 2008, **337**:a258.

64. Koeth RA, Wang Z, Levison BS, et al. **Intestinal microbiota metabolism of l-carnitine, a nutrient in red meat, promotes atherosclerosis.** *Nat Med* 2013.

65. Tang WH, Wang Z, Levison BS, et al. **Intestinal microbial metabolism of phosphatidylcholine and cardiovascular risk.** *N Engl J Med* 2013, **368**:1575-1584.

66. Mozaffarian D, Fahimi S, Singh GM, et al. **Global sodium consumption and death from cardiovascular causes.** *N Engl J Med* 2014, **371**:624-634.

67. Simon G. **Experimental evidence for blood pressure-independent vascular effects of high sodium diet.** *Am J Hypertens* 2003, **16**:1074-1078.

68. Sanders PW. **Vascular consequences of dietary salt intake.** *Am J Physiol Renal Physiol* 2009, **297**:F237-243.

69. Fang J, Cogswell ME, Park S, et al. **Sodium intake among u.s. adults - 26 states, the district of columbia, and puerto rico, 2013.** *MMWR Morb Mortal Wkly Rep* 2015, **64**:695-698.

70. Cook NR, Cutler JA, Obarzanek E, et al. **Long term effects of dietary sodium reduction on cardiovascular disease outcomes: observational follow-up of the trials of hypertension prevention (TOHP).** *BMJ* 2007, **334**:885-888.

71. Bagnardi V, Rota M, Botteri E, et al. **Alcohol consumption and site-specific cancer risk: a comprehensive dose-response meta-analysis.** *Br J Cancer* 2015, **112**:580-593.

72. Saremi A, Arora R. **The cardiovascular implications of alcohol and red wine.** *Am J Ther* 2008, **15**:265-277.

73. Mattes RD, Dreher ML. **Nuts and healthy body weight maintenance mechanisms.** *Asia Pac J Clin Nutr* 2010, **19**:137-141.

74. Levine ME, Suarez JA, Brandhorst S, et al. **Low Protein Intake Is Associated with a Major Reduction in IGF-1, Cancer, and Overall Mortality in the 65 and Younger but Not Older Population.** *Cell Metab* 2014, **19**:407-417.

75. Lagiou P, Sandin S, Lof M, et al. **Low carbohydrate-high protein diet and incidence of cardiovascular diseases in Swedish women: prospective cohort study.** *BMJ* 2012, **344**:e4026.

76. Thissen JP, Ketelslegers JM, Underwood LE. **Nutritional regulation of the insulin-like growth factors.** *Endocr Rev* 1994, **15**:80-101.

77. Kaaks R. **Nutrition, insulin, IGF-1 metabolism and cancer risk: a summary of epidemiological evidence.** *Novartis Found Symp* 2004, **262**:247-260; discussion 260-268.

78. de Oliveira Otto MC, Alonso A, Lee DH, et al. **Dietary intakes of zinc and heme iron from red meat, but not from other sources, are associated with greater risk of metabolic syndrome and cardiovascular disease.** *J Nutr* 2012, **142**:526-533.

79. Yurko-Mauro K, McCarthy D, Rom D, et al. **Beneficial effects of docosahexaenoic acid on cognition in age-related cognitive decline.** *Alzheimers Dement* 2010.

80. Bowman GL, Silbert LC, Howieson D, et al. **Nutrient biomarker patterns, cognitive function, and MRI measures of brain aging.** *Neurology* 2011.

81. Pottala JV, Yaffe K, Robinson JG, et al. **Higher RBC EPA + DHA corresponds with larger total brain and hippocampal volumes: WHIMS-MRI study.** *Neurology* 2014, **82**:435-442.

82. Quinn JF, Raman R, Thomas RG, et al. **Docosahexaenoic acid supplementation and cognitive decline in Alzheimer disease: a randomized trial.** *JAMA* 2010, **304**:1903-1911.

83. **Environmental Working Group. PCBs in farmed salmon.** [http://www.ewg.org/research/pcbs-farmed-salmon]

84. **EPA-FDA Advisory on mercury in fish and shellfish** [https://www.epa.gov/fish-tech/epa-fda-advisory-mercury-fish-and-shellfish]

85. **Office of Dietary Supplements, National Institutes of Health. Dietary supplement fact sheet: vitamin B12** [http://ods.od.nih.gov/factsheets/VitaminB12/]

86. Mozos I, Marginean O. **Links between Vitamin D Deficiency and Cardiovascular Diseases.** *Biomed Res Int* 2015, **2015**:109275.

87. Holick MF. **Sunlight and vitamin D for bone health and prevention of autoimmune diseases, cancers, and cardiovascular disease.** *Am J Clin Nutr* 2004, **80**:1678S-1688S.

88. Kidd PM. **Vitamins D and K as pleiotropic nutrients: clinical importance to the skeletal and cardiovascular systems and preliminary evidence for synergy.** *Altern Med Rev* 2010, **15**:199-222.

89. Rees K, Guraewal S, Wong YL, et al. **Is vitamin K consumption associated with cardio-metabolic disorders? A systematic review.** *Maturitas* 2010, **67**:121-128.

90. Beulens JW, Bots ML, Atsma F, et al. **High dietary menaquinone intake is associated with reduced coronary calcification.** *Atherosclerosis* 2009, **203**:489-493.

91. **Office of Dietary Supplements, National Institutes of Health. Dietary supplement fact sheet: iodine.**

92. **Office of Dietary Supplements, National Institutes of Health. Dietary supplement fact sheet: zinc.** [http://ods.od.nih.gov/factsheets/Zinc-HealthProfessional/]

93. Hunt JR. **Bioavailability of iron, zinc, and other trace minerals from vegetarian diets.** *Am J Clin Nutr* 2003, **78**:633S-639S.

94. Bjelakovic G, Nikolova D, Gluud C. **Meta-regression analyses, meta-analyses, and trial sequential analyses of the effects of supplementation with beta-carotene, vitamin A, and vitamin singly or in different combinations on all-cause mortality: do we have evidence for lack of harm?** *PLoS One* 2013, **8**:e74558.

95. Bjelakovic G, Nikolova D, Gluud LL, et al. **Antioxidant supplements for prevention of mortality in healthy participants and patients with various diseases.** *Cochrane Database Syst Rev* 2008:CD007176.

96. Brewer GJ. **Risks of copper and iron toxicity during aging in humans.** *Chem Res Toxicol* 2010, **23**:319-326.

97. Smith AD, Kim YI, Refsum H. **Is folic acid good for everyone?** *Am Clin Nutr* 2008, **87**:517-533.

98. Ebbing M, Bonaa KH, Nygard O, et al. **Cancer incidence and mortality after treatment with folic acid and vitamin B12.** *JAMA* 2009, **302**:2119-2126.

99. Swanson D, Block R, Mousa SA. **Omega-3 fatty acids EPA and DHA: health benefits throughout life.** *Adv Nutr* 2012, **3**:1-7.

100. Kris-Etherton PM, Harris WS, Appel LJ, Association AHANCAH. **Omega-3 fatty acids and cardiovascular disease: new recommendations from the American Heart Association.** *Arterioscler Thromb Vasc Biol* 2003, **23**:151-152.

101. Harris WS. **The omega-3 index as a risk factor for coronary heart disease.** *Am J Clin Nutr* 2008, **87**:1997S-2002S.

102. Musa-Veloso K, Binns MA, Kocenas A, et al. **Impact of low v. moderate intakes of long-chain n-3 fatty acids on risk of coronary heart disease.** *Br J Nutr* 2011.

103. Alexander DD, Miller PE, Van Elswyk ME, et al. **A meta-analysis of randomized controlled trials and prospective cohort studies of eicosapentaenoic and docosahexaenoic long-chain omega-fatty acids and coronary heart disease risk.** *Mayo Clin Proc* 2017, **92**:15-29.

104. Burr ML. **Secondary prevention of CHD in UK men: the Diet and Reinfarction Trial and its sequel.** *Proc Nutr Soc* 2007, **66**:9-15.

105. Ras RT, Geleijnse JM, Trautwein EA. **LDL-cholesterol-lowering effect of plant sterols and stanols across different dose ranges a meta-analysis of randomised controlled studies.** *Br J Nutr* 2014, **112**:214-219.

106. Wang ZM, Zhou B, Wang YS, et al. **Black and green tea consumption and the risk of coronary artery disease: a meta-analysis.** *The American journal of clinical nutrition* 2011, **93**:506-515.

107. Onakpoya I, Spencer E, Heneghan C, Thompson M. **The effect of green tea on blood pressure and lipid profile: a systematic review and meta-analysis of randomized clinical trials.** *Nutr Metab Cardiovasc Dis* 2014, **24**:823-836.

108. Panahi Y, Hosseini MS, Khalili N, et al. **Antioxidant and anti-inflammatory effects of curcuminoid-piperine combination in subjects with metabolic syndrome: A randomized controlled trial and an updated meta-analysis.** *Clin Nutr* 2015, **34**:1101-1108

109. Sahebkar A. **Are curcuminoids effective C-reactive protein-lowering agents in clinical practice? Evidence from a meta-analysis.** *Phytother Res* 2014, **28**:633-642.49. Fan J, Song Y, Wang Y, et al. **Dietary glycemic index, glycemic load, and risk of coronary heart disease, stroke, and stroke mortality: a systematic review with meta-analysis.** *PLoS One* 2012, **7**:e52182.